She was tall and slender. Her golden hair was pinned up loosely in a bun. Her breasts were firm and round, featuring long nipples that pointed toward the sky. Her skin was silky smooth, her eyes deep blue, and her lips a burgundy red.

She scurried to the limo, her breasts slightly jiggled with her every move. The chauffeur opened the door for her and she slid into the backseat. Ken greeted her with a kiss on her cheek and a glass of champagne. He was taking her to the opera.

He lifted her hand and placed a kiss on each of her fingers. Then he placed one in his mouth deliberately and sucked gently on it. Turning her hand, he placed a light kiss at the base of her wrist. He grinned and moved closer so that he could nibble at her earlobe. She shivered a bit, even though it wasn't cold. He nibbled his way down her neck to where her breasts parted.

COME QUICKLY:
For Couples on the Go

JULIAN ANTHONY GUERRA, EDITOR

MASQUERADE BOOKS, INC.
801 SECOND AVENUE
NEW YORK, N.Y. 10017

First Masquerade Edition 1996

First Printing December 1996

ISBN 1-56333-461-5

Manufactured in the United States of America
Published by Masquerade Books, Inc.
801 Second Avenue
New York, N.Y. 10017

COME QUICKLY

Preface

I'm gonna make this fast. And you're gonna like it! What we've got here are a few dozen quickies. One-handed reading for the Evelyn Wood crowd. Something nice and hot and juicy. Something for you to enjoy on the john in your office bathroom during your coffee break. We all know why we're here. Why bother with the elaborate setup? Let's just cut to the chase and get sweaty!

That's what *Come Quickly* is all about. Most of the writers here are new. A few have written in earlier Masquerade anthologies. The one thing I asked of all of them is, use as few words as possible to turn me on as fast as they can. Well, let me tell you something: I gave each of these stories a test drive, and boy, am I sore!

So forget the cologne, the fancy dinner, and the nightcap. Just turn the page, sit back for a moment, and enjoy. Once in a while it feels good to say, "Fuck it!" And come quickly....

Julian Anthony Guerra
Editor

BEST OF FRIENDS
Claire Watson

Joanie and Erica loved toying with Bobby. Teasing him about his new haircut, they circled around him, tickling his neck and pulling on his earlobes. He knew them too well. They had plenty of potential for getting quite obnoxious, but he loved it when they touched him.

Both were gorgeous. Erica was tall and slim with short champagne-blond hair. She had almond-shaped blue eyes, long, muscular limbs, and tiny but firm breasts. Joanie was a little shorter than Erica. Her dark brown hair was long and curly. She had large brown eyes, rounded hips and full, round breasts.

They'd been friends since kindergarten, and in recent years, they'd gotten quite a reputation for being the biggest cockteases. Of course, Bobby didn't care. He enjoyed everything about them. He liked their looks, their smell, the way they giggled when they thought they'd embarrassed him. He even liked the way they would look at each other exchanging some secret method of communication that only friends as close as they were could have developed.

Today they were flirting with him because they wanted a ride home. He was more than happy to oblige, but wasn't going to make it easy for them.

"I'll give you a lift, but you'd better behave yourselves!" he warned them.

"Behave? What on earth do you mean? We're good girls!" Erica whined.

"Yeah, well, we'll see about that. Get in."

Giggling again, they jumped in the backseat. He had become their chauffeur.

"Drive on, Bobby," Erica ordered, while Joanie giggled.

He couldn't focus on the road. He kept looking at them in his rearview mirror. Joanie had slipped her hand under Erica's blouse and started massaging her breasts. They were staring into each other's eyes, knowing full well that their chauffeur's face was turning red with nervousness and excitement. He didn't know what to do with himself.

Erica tilted Joanie's head upward and gave her a long and gentle French kiss. Joanie continued to work on Erica's breasts, pinching and pulling her small, hard pink nipples. Erica slowly pulled off her tank top, and continued to kiss Joanie. Joanie decided she wanted her top off as well, and made quite a show of wiggling out of it.

Their bodies were different, but equally exquisite. They rubbed their tits together, feeling each other's hard nipples. They were really gazing at each other now, their eyes glazed over with passion. They'd done this many times and clearly knew how to please one another.

Joanie pulled up her pleated miniskirt and spread her legs. Bobby gasped when he saw that she wasn't wearing any panties. He started to stroke his massive hard-on through his jeans while trying to drive straight.

Erica inserted two fingers into Joanie's dripping cunt. With her thumb, she massaged Joanie's clit. Erica gave Joanie her breasts to nibble on while she was being finger-fucked.

The smell of their juices wafted into the front seat. Bobby wanted to touch them, lick them, and hopefully fuck them so badly. He pulled over to the side and turned the engine off.

"I thought I told you to behave yourselves. Not only are you being naughty, but rude, too! You didn't even invite me!"

"Oh, poor Bobby—he feels left out!" Joanie's voice dripped with sweet sarcasm.

"We thought you didn't want to be bothered," Erica added.

"I told you to behave, and decent behavior would be to include your host in the party!"

"Hmm. Well, since we're at the bargaining table, Joanie and I would like to know what else you have to offer besides a ride home?"

"How about this!"

Bobby unzipped his stonewashed jeans and pulled out his long, thick cock. It had a large, wide head, and it already glistened with precome. The girls' eyes widened with lust. They smiled and reached for Bobby's proud offering.

They reached over and grabbed his cock, pulling him around to face them. Joanie handled his shaft and head while Erica inspected his balls.

"I wanna suck it." Joanie looked at him and licked her lips.

"Age before beauty," Erica sniped.

Joanie sneered at her girlfriend, and then leaned down in front of Bobby's cock, taking the whole thing in her mouth. She sucked hard and fast while holding his ass tightly, digging her nails into his firm cheeks.

Erica sat in the backseat and positioned herself in front of Joanie's ass. She pulled Joanie's asscheeks apart and licked her girlfriend's little pink hole. She then started to finger-fuck Joanie's wet cunt. Joanie began to go wild.

Erica pulled her jeans down and started playing with her clit.

"I can't hold out any longer—I think I'm gonna come!" The sight of these two horny girls, sucking him and playing with one another brought Bobby closer and closer to climax.

"Fuck her mouth, Bobby! And when you're ready, let me swallow your come!" Erica whispered.

He held Joanie's head and fucked her mouth deep, virtually hitting the back of her throat, but Joanie was accommodating him with no problem. Her cunt was soaked. She was gyrating her hips, pushing her ass into Erica's hungry tongue. Erica fucked Joanie faster and harder until Joanie exploded into orgasm. Her screams of ecstasy were muffled by Bobby's cock.

"Erica, get ready—I'm coming!"

Erica moved closer to Bobby, opened her mouth, and stuck her tongue out for him. He moved his leaping cock onto her tongue and spilled his come in long, drawn-out spurts. Soon her mouth was full. She closed her lips around his fat head and sucked it until there was nothing left. She felt her tongue and the back of her throat tingle as she swallowed his jism.

Bobby sighed with relief and smiled at the two of them.

"Can you please take us home now?" Joanie asked.

"I'll take you wherever you wanna go!" Bobby was leaning back against the dashboard, completely out of breath.

"Just drive on, Bobby—while I make sure that Erica gets off, now that she's been fed!"

They both smiled at him from the backseat and went back to what they'd started before their *chauffeur* had interrupted them so plaintively.

PIANO LESSONS
Jason McDermott

He was glad he'd chosen his baggy black trousers to wear
today because his cock was getting harder by the minute.
He was concentrating on her long, lean legs rather than
her fingers. She was stroking the ivory keys of the baby
grand, moving her body to the rhythm of the song.

Her plush chestnut hair was pulled in a tight bun,
accentuating her long, smooth neck. Her skin was soft
and pale, which made her dark eyes and full red lips look
quite dramatic. Her breasts were small, but her nipples
were pushing through her silky white blouse. He was
fixated on her thighs, watching the right one move up
and down without skipping a beat.

She stopped playing, looked at him, and told him to
repeat what she had just finished playing.

"I'm not sure I can," he replied earnestly.

"Do your best, and if you get stuck I'll guide you," she answered with a smile.

With a slight awkwardness he began pounding on the keys.

"Gently," she whispered. She took a hold of his hand and held it between her palms.

"Pretend that the piano is a sensitive woman. One who needs to be caressed."

She stared into his dark brown eyes and slowly pulled his hands to her lips. Without breaking her gaze, she began to lick his fingertips.

Suddenly his cock felt like it was going to explode. She reached down between his legs and rubbed the bulge firmly.

"You must learn to feel the music with your body and soul," she whispered.

She raised her left leg over the piano stool and spread her thighs wide open. She brought his wet fingers to her pussy and started to stroke herself with his hand.

"Now play!"

To his surprise, he realized that she wasn't wearing panties. He pushed two fingers inside her, feeling the warm, juicy flesh of her cunt. She unbuttoned her blouse, exposing her small, firm breasts with her large brown, hard nipples.

"Suck on them."

He bent forward and drew her left nipple into his mouth. He sucked long and hard, listening to her moan in response. He alternated from one nipple to the other.

"Now I want to return the favor," she smiled.

His teacher knelt at the foot of the bench, unzipped his pants, and pulled out his thick, turgid cock. Her long fingers surrounded the shaft and she pushed down on it while squeezing firmly, forcing the blood to rush to the head. A soft, almost helpless groan signified he could help himself no longer. He grabbed the back of her head, pushing it on his swollen meat.

With the tip of her tongue, she teased him, forcing him to grow bigger still. Suddenly she shoved the whole thing down her throat, sucking on it with an enthusiasm that bordered on fury. Her body was now moving to the beat of her throat being fucked. She was like a wild, hungry animal. She straddled his leg and rubbed her juicy pussy on it, bringing her to a higher state of ecstasy.

She reached up under his shirt and found one of his nipples. She pinched it and pulled on it as she continued to make a meal out of his throbbing prick. His body tensed. He took her head and held it tight as his dick jolted as far down into her throat as it could possibly go. Finally he began to spasm, shooting load after load inside her mouth. She swallowed as much as she could, while the rest oozed from the edges of her glossy lips.

He pulled her up and kissed her come-filled mouth, shoving his tongue inside and sucking his leftover juices from her.

"You did well this time," she grinned. "Not bad for a second lesson. For your third lesson, we will study the key of G Major."

BIRTHDAY PRESENT
Patty Thorn

Sylvia knew that Nathan was up to something, and that made her nervous with excitement. He always came up with the most creative ways to celebrate her birthdays.

She was an elegant woman. Tall, slender, long auburn hair and almond-shaped hazel eyes. Her skin was alabaster, as soft as satin.

Today she was wearing a long black silk dress with spaghetti straps and her high-heeled patent-leather sandals. She decided to accessorize with the pearl choker that Nathan gave her for her last birthday. Dabbed with a spicy perfume behind her ears and on her wrists, she was ready to celebrate.

"Honey, whenever you're ready come down!" Nate called up from the living room.

Sylvia stole a glance in the mirror one last time. Satisfied with what she saw she made her way downstairs to meet her husband.

All the lights were turned off. There were scented candles and dozens of red roses everywhere. In the background she could hear music playing.

She looked around for Nathan, but he wasn't in sight. After relaxing on the couch for a few minutes with a glass of wine, she felt a hand touch her bare shoulder.

"Don't turn around," he whispered very softly in her ear. "Close your eyes and breathe deeply."

He gently stroked her hair, then her neck, and he kissed her ears, thrilling to her spicy scent. Slipping his large hands down her low-cut dress, he tweaked her nipples until they hardened. She pushed her torso forward, wanting more. He leaned over and kissed her lips, just as she opened her eyes to look at him.

She jumped in shock. *This man was not her husband!*

He smiled at her surprise.

"Who are you?"

"I'm your birthday present, Sylvia." His voice was warm and deep.

"Don't worry, hon, I'm right here. You always said you'd like to have two men at the same time. Happy birthday!"

Sylvia didn't know what to say. She looked at both of them, and then, with only a single moment's hesitation, gave her husband the biggest smile.

"Well, thank you very much!" she leaned over and kissed her husband. "I think I'll play with my present now. What's your name?"

"Mike."

"Nice to meet you, Mike." She flipped her straps of her shoulders and let her dress fall to her ankles. She casually stepped over her dress, to sit back down on the couch in only her shoes and pearl necklace. There, she spread her legs wide.

"Eat my pussy, Mike."

"My pleasure, Sylvia."

He kneeled between her legs and began to lick her wet pink pussy. He probed her with his tongue and slipped a finger in her tight asshole. She threw her head back, breathing deeply, a delicate sheen of perspiration already causing her flesh to glow.

"I want your cock in my mouth, Nate." She licked her finger and gazed at her husband.

In no time, he dropped his clothes, hopped on the couch next to her, and fed her his hard-on. She took hold of it, stuffing it in her mouth as if she'd been starved. She loved sucking dick, and he knew it.

Mike stood up and removed his clothes. He was muscular and tan. His dick was enormous. He stroked it several times, feeling it grow hard as he watched Nathan face-fuck Sylvia. He sat next to her and played with her nipples. It wouldn't be long before she let go of Nate's dick and turned to Mike.

"I want to sit on your dick, Mike."

"Just say the word, Sylvia." His smile was warm in the soft candlelight of the living room.

She propped herself over his massive dick and sat on it, feeling her pussy stretch the farther down she slid. She moaned with pleasure and began to ride him.

"Fuck my ass, Nathan."

"Whatever you say, babe."

She leaned forward, giving Nathan easy access to her ass. Mike took the opportunity to stuff his face with her tits. He suckled on them, making her tremble. Nathan spat on his fingers and inserted them in her asshole for lubrication. He worked that tight hole until he felt her relax. Only then did he pull her cheeks apart and push his dick slowly inside. Her whole body quivered, and a squeal of delight escaped her lips.

Mike nibbled on her nipples while she rode him violently. Nate was fucking her ass slow and hard. Her body began to spasm, and her pussy flooded Mike's dick with its juices. With a guttural scream, she continued to bounce on him, driving her orgasm to new heights. Nathan grabbed Sylvia's hair and pulled her head back. He fucked her ass faster and faster.

"Fuck me, Nate! Fuck me!" she was yelling.

"I'm coming, babe!" Nate gasped back. "I'm coming!"

He felt her pussy muscles contract around his dick, and it was as if her sweet box was sucking his cock. He pushed up into her, and in seconds he exploded inside her.

He spilled his come deep in her asshole, and stayed inside her until he had nothing more left. As he pulled out, some of his come oozed out of her snatch and dripped down her thighs.

The three of them sat together with Sylvia in the middle. They hugged and kissed and she gently stroked their dicks.

"Happy birthday!" The two men said in unison.

"This was the best birthday yet. Now I think I'll make a wish—and then I'll blow." She smiled and winked at the two of them. The night had just begun!

SQUEAKY CLEAN
Peter Sheldon

6:00 A.M. in the gym's sauna. No one there except the two of us. Her towel came off, and she asked me to massage her. "I'm so sore from the workout," she said.

I began to rub her shoulders, moving slowly down to her lower back. Her muscles were tight.

"Relax. I'll work out the kinks."

"Thanks, I really needed this."

We'd worked out many times together, spotting each other, exchanging exercise tips. We had become quite friendly. I guess she felt comfortable enough with me.

She was quite a knockout: tall, muscular, with large, round breasts, firm buttocks, tight tummy, and an even tan. She had thick shoulder-length hair, streaked with blonde. Her nails were long and always polished, and she wore expensive perfumes. If she only knew the perverse thoughts I'd been having about her, she probably wouldn't come near me.

So there she was, naked in the sauna, asking me to massage her smooth, strong back. This was a dream come true! Her tits were succulent. Her nipples looked like pencil erasers. Her pussy was neatly shaved, exposing her luscious thick lips. I started rubbing her neck and shoulders, worried because my dick was growing bigger by the second.

"Wow! I think I need a cold shower," I told her, trying to save myself from embarrassment.

"What a great idea! I think I'll join you," she replied. "But I want a warm shower, not a cold one."

As we got up, she noticed my tremendous hard-on. I didn't know what to do with myself.

"I take it *this* is why you want a cold shower." She smiled.

I nodded weakly.

"That would be a waste, don't you think?" And with that question she grabbed my dick tightly and led me into the showers.

"It's a good thing the place is empty at this time. Now I want that massage you promised. I'd be glad to return the favor."

She turned on the shower and adjusted the temperature of the water. The warm water splashed over our bodies.

Then she braced my dick with both her hands and began to masturbate me. I was dizzy with excitement.

"Now stick your cock inside me and massage my cunt with it."

She leaned back on the tiled wall for support. I lifted her leg and let it rest over my arm, exposing her hungry cunt. With cock in hand, I searched for her clit. Once I found it, I massaged it, as promised, with my thick cock-head. Her cunt was soaked, and it was more than just the water from the shower. Slowly, I forced my fat cock into her tight cunt, stretching it wider the deeper I went.

I pushed my body up against hers, thrilling to the feel of her hard nipples poking into my torso. I leaned down and stuck my tongue in her mouth, sucking on her tongue as I chewed on her lips. Her breathing had gotten heavy and fast. I fucked her hard, slamming her body into the wall with every thrust. I knew that after I was through, she was gonna have a sore pussy. She was getting the massage of her life!

Now she was digging her nails into my back. It made me want to fuck her even harder. I licked and sucked at her neck as I fucked her, and she began to moan louder and louder. She pulled her hips forward and shuddered. I put all my body weight up against hers and rammed my cock fast and furious, until I exploded inside that hot, throbbing pussy of hers.

I stayed, leaning against her for a little longer, feeling the warm water splashing on my back. Her firm, wet body felt so damned good! I think I'll become her personal masseur. No charge!

STEPMOM
Tony Gould

When Dad introduced me to the woman who would soon be his bride, I was beside myself! Not only was she too young for him, but she was drop-dead gorgeous. For the first time in my life, I was jealous of my own father.

After a few weeks, when it finally sank in that this chick was going to be living in my home and telling me what to do, my evil eighteen-year-old mind began to focus on the advantages. This was going to be an enjoyable live-in situation.

She was a fun stepmom. As I got to know her, I really began to enjoy her company. She'd often point out that we had so much in common, but she'd also say there was a lot I needed to learn. I wondered what she meant. Better yet, I hoped that she was planning to teach me!

The day came when the situation was right, and she decided it was time for my lesson.

"Tommy, have you ever seen a woman naked?"

"Not really," I answered with what must have been a stupid grin, my ears burning. "I mean, not all the way in real life. Plenty of times in *Playboy.*"

"I think it's time for you to see what a woman looks like," she said matter-of-factly.

She began to strip. I was in shock. My fantasies about her just vaporized at that moment, and all I could think about was my father walking in on us.

"Relax, Tommy. You have nothing to worry about. Your dad won't be home until tomorrow night. He's got a business meeting out of town."

Her body was perfect. She had long smooth legs, a flat stomach, a well-trimmed pussy, a full, firm ass, and large, pointy breasts. Her nipples were long and thick and stuck straight out. I was salivating mentally—I got an instant hard-on!

She looked at me and smiled, "Now, Tommy I don't want you to be nervous. Clearly, there are some things you must learn, and I'm willing to teach you."

I hadn't lied to her. I'd had more than a few girl-friends in the past, and had gotten pretty far with them. It would have been only a matter of time before my cherry was popped. But I certainly wasn't going to deny her a crack at this "teaching" trip!

"I want you to take off all of your clothes and sit next to me on the bed," she instructed.

My dick was standing at attention. I followed her

orders to the letter. She slipped her hand around my shaft and stroked my head with her thumb. I thought I was going to explode right then and there, but I breathed in deeply, thought about baseball, and tried to maintain control.

"You have such a large penis, Tommy. It's so thick and long. I would just love to taste it! Would that be okay with you?"

"I guess so," I managed to mumble.

She kneeled in front of my erection and rolled her tongue around the rim of my cock. Catching the head in her luscious lips, she slid all the way down my shaft, taking me in like no other girl had ever done. She then began to suck wildly, pushing me back and forth and digging her nails into my buttcheeks. I felt weird and crazy, standing there, being devoured by my stepmom—but it felt so good!

I was almost ready to come when she stopped. She stood up and wiped her mouth. She stood so close to me, I could feel her nipples poking into my chest. She was slightly taller, and that just added to the incestuous feeling.

"You have excellent control, Tommy. That's very important to a woman."

"I'm going to lie on the bed, and I want you to lie next to me. I'm going to show you how to play with a woman's pussy."

We lay next to each other, and she spread her legs. She took my hand and guided it to her wet, hungry cunt. It was soft, warm, and juicy.

"Stroke my clit, gently and slowly at first. Then you can increase the speed and the intensity of your touch."

I obliged her by following her instructions carefully. Her soft moans and groans made me feel good, as if I was being a good student. She began stroking my cock, as I moved my fingers over her clit more quickly. She started to lift and turn her hips, taking the pleasure I was giving her.

"Fuck me, Tommy—I think you're ready now!"

I jumped on top of her and rammed my dick into her hungry cunt. I fucked her hard and fast while sucking on her nipples. She'd started screaming and clawing my back—less a stepmom or a teacher, and more like an animal—and I was feeding her with my massive cock.

"Fuck me harder, Tommy! Fuck me till I'm sore!"

I wasn't going to let her down. I grabbed onto her hair and ramrodded her pussy forcefully. She was rolling her head from side to side, pushing her hips up. Her body tensed. Her groans became guttural. She screamed and shook, and I felt her cunt contract around my dick.

"Oh, Tommy!" she gasped. "That was great! You're such a good student!"

She kissed me deeply as I continued to fuck her, gently pinching and pulling on my nipples, again, like no girl I'd been with had ever done. I couldn't hold back any longer.

"Come, baby, come for Mama!"

I gave her ten final strokes and shot my load with such force, I thought my balls would implode!

I fell limp on her body breathing heavily resting my face on her sweaty tits.

"That was your first lesson." She grinned. "You're going to be such an excellent student. Of course, there's going to be plenty of homework!"

My stepmom was going to be very proud of me. I had every intention of being class valedictorian!

SWEETS FOR THE SWEET
Philip Woll

She smeared chocolate fudge between her palms and rubbed it all over my hard cock, massaging the shaft until it was completely covered with the warm, sticky goo. Looking into my eyes she took the head of my dick into her hot mouth and began feasting on my candied tool. The sweetness made her salivate, slicking the meat, forcing her to wolf it down like the glutton for cock she was.

I'd always known she couldn't resist chocolate. This was the best idea I'd had in months! Taking my balls into her hands, she massaged them between her palms. I felt her finger find my asshole with ease, and she proceeded to enter my hole without hesitation. I almost cried out, but she made it feel so damned good!

My dick was hard and ready to explode inside her

mouth. She must have read my mind, because she pulled away and gave me a sly smile.

"You're not coming now, are you? I'm not done with you yet!" She scooped out some more chocolate fudge and dressed my aching dick with it. She carefully coated every inch, including my balls. I couldn't bear this torture for much longer.

I felt her luscious lips on the head of my chocolate-dipped dick and helped her to a second serving. She licked my shaft up and down and then she went for my balls. She popped each one into her mouth, like bonbons, cleaning them thoroughly with her tongue and letting them drop out when all the chocolate was gone.

"I think I'm full now." She smiled up at me.

"That's what you think! You're not done until I say so, Little Miss Sweet Tooth! Now open wide, and don't forget to swallow!"

Without hesitation, I knelt over her face and aimed my fat, hard dick into her chocolate-smeared mouth. She almost looked worried, but there was more sugar yet to come.

"Now suck real nice, and you'll get a real treat!"

I started pumping her head, feeling her tongue and teeth scrape my thick meat. My heart was racing, and I could hear her muffled moans. I couldn't tell whether she was in pleasure or pain; but as long as her lips and tongue were skillfully doing their job, I knew she was fine.

Her lips tightened around my dick and her tongue swirled around the shaft. Soon I couldn't control myself any longer. With a fierce thrust, I spilled my come inside her mouth in a series of waves that had my head spinning! But I didn't pull out!

"Suck it, baby. Suck it dry and swallow it. This stuff is a helluva lot better than your chocolate goo!"

I felt her cheeks and throat contract as she swallowed every last bit of my jism, even while her mouth was still stuffed with my dick. She held the tip delicately between her fingers after I finally pulled out, licking every last drop. She looked up at me and showed me her pearly whites. I knew she was finally satiated.

"Next week," I told her, "marshmallow fluff!"

THE HITCHHIKER
Butch Anheimer

"Hey, where are you headed?" she asked the stranger behind the wheel of the white Cutlass Supreme.

"I'm going west."

"Great! That's exactly where I wanna be!"

"Well, hop on in," he grinned.

She flung her duffel bag in the back and plopped her petite round ass on the leather seat.

Her firm, smooth legs and thighs were tanned and dappled with golden peach fuzz that rose to meet the frayed hem of her denim shorts. Her tight baby-blue undershirt caressed her small pointy breasts, and her fine strawberry-blonde hair tickled her sun-browned shoulders.

"You're a brave young girl," he commented as he put the car in gear.

"I like adventure, and my instincts have never failed me." She sounded confident, almost perky.

"Well I'm glad I found some company," he glanced at her before looking out at the road. "Driving alone either makes me tense or sleepy."

"I think I know how to keep you awake and relaxed." She pulled off her undershirt, looked into his eyes, and tweaked her large dark nipples gently. "Pull off at the next exit."

By the time he'd pulled off the road and coasted the car up to some brush, her shorts were already off and her ass was sticking up at him, eagerly awaiting his next move. He unzipped his pants and pulled out his cock.

"Fuck my ass!" she yelled, as she slapped her left buttcheek. He bent down and stuck his tongue up her tight asshole. She moaned in ecstasy as he moistened her hole as deeply as his tongue could reach. When she was well lubricated with his spit, he pulled her cheeks wide apart and inserted his middle finger into her pink butthole. Sighing, she pushed into him. He then slid his index finger into the fleshy chute and twisted his hand as he pulled it in and out.

"Fuck me!" She was shouting at him now. "I don't wan wait any more."

"No problem, baby!"

He grabbed her hair and jerked her head backward, forcing her to look up. He poked her ass with his stiff cock until his swollen head found her burning little hole. He forced his way in slowly, pushing and stretching her lubricated asshole. Her guttural moans gave him a rush, inspiring him to fuck her harder and faster. She reached between her legs to rub her clit furiously, her juices oozing down the insides of her thighs. She searched for his balls with her pussy-wet fingers; and when she found them, she cupped them and massaged them, causing him to fuck her with even more vigor.

Squeezing her clit between her thumb and forefinger, she pulled, pinched, and rubbed it until her whole body started to quake into orgasm after orgasm.

With both his hands on her waist, he pulled her ass into him with greater and greater force, slapping her cheeks with his hips. Her wildly rotating hips helped to pull and push his shaft until he finally exploded, filling her up with his thick come.

He held her tight as his body relaxed, and he leaned down on her to catch his breath, feeling her sweaty back on his torso.

"I think our trip out west will take a bit longer than I expected," he whispered in her ear before licking and chewing at her lobe.

"Sorry, guy." The sweaty blonde hitchhiker smiled back. "Ride's over. Gotta be movin' on to the next luxury car. You might say I'm a collector!"

THE SHOE SALESMAN
Jack Tobie

Mario was closing the store, but Angie begged him to let her in. She'd come to Shoe Heaven knowing exactly which pair of shoes she needed, and she would be only five minutes. How could he refuse?

Mario located the red patent leather stiletto heels in her size, but they were too narrow. Her toes ached.

"I'll make them feel better," Mario said.

"Wait! What the hell are you doing?"

"Look—you're tired. I see you've been running around all day. Just let me do this for you," Mario said, rather matter-of-factly. "Gimme one minute. Sixty seconds. If you don't like it, I'll give you the shoes free of charge."

"Free? Just try it. You got sixty."

He placed his lips on her throbbing toes and sucked them through her nylon stockings. A moan escaped her lips, despite herself. He tore the sheer nylons and sucked on each toe individually. Her shock at his behavior was tempered by the incredible sensations traveling from the tips of her toes to the suddenly throbbing center of her clit.

She closed her eyes, leaned back on the black vinyl chair and relaxed her legs. With the other foot, she searched for his chest. His shirt was buttoned all the way to the top and secured with a maroon-and-gold-striped silk necktie. She rubbed her foot over and under his tie searching for a way to find bare skin. Realizing her desires, he quickly loosened a couple of buttons, giving her easy access to his hairy torso.

The curls of his chest hairs sent electric tingling sensations through her sole into the depths of his stomach. Holding her right foot, he massaged it gently with his warm hands while licking and nibbling on her meaty heel. He traced her deep arch with his tongue until he reached her small, plump toes. With great relish, he sucked each one into his mouth twirling his tongue between them.

"My minute's up." Mario smiled. "Should I go on?"

"No!" Angie gasped. "Uh, waitaminnit! Yes!"

He could smell the sweet aroma of her wet pussy mingling with the scent of the red patent-leather shoes. He looked up at her to see her playing with her nipples over her mint-colored satin shirt. They must be large ones he thought to himself. Maybe as large as her little toe. With that thought, he sucked harder on her little toe, making her moan louder and spread her legs as wide as the store chair would allow. He noticed that she wasn't wearing any panties. Her pubic hair was kept neatly in place covered by her pantyhose.

"I want you to play with my clit," she pleaded softly to him. "But don't stop massaging my feet."

With her foot inside his mouth, he reached between her thighs and traced her pussylips with his finger through her torn pantyhose.

She shuddered slightly, barely able to catch her breath.

He tore a larger hole in the crotch of her pantyhose, giving him direct access to her clit. He probed through only to touch a warm, wet, throbbing, hard knob. He thought his dick would explode right then and there. Still sucking on her toes, he took a deep breath and started flicking her clit with his thumb.

Her moans turned into short, breathy grunts. She had tilted her head all the way back. Her hips were now off the chair. She was balancing herself on the arms of the seat, with her feet propped against his mouth and chest.

"Ma'am? would it be acceptable to you if I played with myself?" Mario asked with the utmost respect.

"Yes. Just make sure you keep one hand on my pussy!"

"Thank you, ma'am. I'll do anything you like. At Shoe Heaven we always please our customers."

He pulled out his thick, hard dick and stroked it

slowly, squeezing it as tightly as he could. She looked down at him holding and stroking himself that way, and suddenly had the urge to feel the texture of his hard dick on the bottom of her feet. She lowered them from his chest, down his tummy, and under his thick shaft. She sandwiched his balls with both her feet and pressed gently.

"Move your hand away from your dick," she ordered.

Without hesitation, he obliged.

She inched her toes upward, pushing his dick against his body. She could almost see his heart racing in his chest.

"I'm gonna make you come!" With that, she began to rub her feet up and down his shaft, shoving it against him. His thumb continued to flick at her clit, and she plucked at her own nipples, thrilling to the feeling of his pulsating meat.

"Ma'am, I can't hold off anymore. May I please have permission to come?"

"Not until I come first!"

He felt ashamed that he had been so selfish. He reached out and stroked her calves gently. He moved up behind her knees and ran his fingers up and down the back of her long, lean legs. That seemed to do the trick.

Her body began to shake, and her grunts turned into a long, loud tone of ecstasy. Her pussyjuices oozed between her fingers down the crack of her ass forming a small glistening pool on the seat of the black vinyl chair.

"May I come now, ma'am?" Mario was pleading now.

"Yes, I want to feel your come on my feet!"

Angie pushed and stroked his dick as hard as she could. He palmed her ankles, helping her to move her feet up and down until, with a sudden burst, his come exploded from the head of his cock, shooting up onto his chest.

At last he sighed with relief and looked her in the eyes.

She gave him half a smile and without a moment to waste, she used her feet to massage the come all over his hairy chest.

"Now, clean my feet with your tongue," said Angie, lost in the power of it all. "And don't miss a spot!"

"With pleasure, ma'am."

"And when you're done, don't forget to wrap my shoes."

"Yes, ma'am! Will that be cash or charge?"

ROMEO DU JOUR
Olga Mathersby

Sue finally reached home, dripping wet from the heavy rain. Her stockings were positively plastered to her thighs, and her black high heels were caked with mud. After a long, stressful day at work, what she really needed was some peace and quiet, and a hot meal. Searching through a file folder stuffed with menus, she realized that most takeout joints had stopped delivering a half an hour ago.

Romeo's was one that was still open. Their service was usually pretty good, and the Italian food was passable.

The phone rang several times before the man answered with an annoyed tone in his voice.

"I'd like to order a Sicilian pie with pepperoni and a diet Coke to be delivered." Enough for tonight and the next few days, she thought. A fair-enough deal.

"You're in luck, I was just about to shut down. Let me have your address and phone number."

Before she knew it, the doorbell was chiming.

"Who's there?"

"Delivery from Romeo's."

She buzzed the delivery person while checking her pocketbook for cash.

The delivery boy turned out to be a tall, stocky dark-haired man in his late-twenties. Raindrops glistened in his thick chestnut locks. He seemed somewhat annoyed.

"How much?" she asked.

"Twelve dollars."

"Do you have change for a fifty?"

"Are you joking? I don't have that kind of change!"

"Oh. Well, I'm sorry, but this is all I have. Is there any way that I can make it up to you?

Assessing her from head to toe, he cracked the slightest hint of a smile. He stepped into her apartment, placed the pizza on an end table, and started opening his slicker.

"C'mon, lady. A girl like you who could afford an apartment like this ought to have as much as I need between the cushions in your couch!"

"Well, I'm not about to go searching!" He'd have been obnoxious if it weren't for that twinkle in his eye. He was kinda cute. "Tell you what. You look a little chilly. Why don't I try to warm you up?"

"Well," he shrugged and sniffed. "That sounds like it might be a fair trade."

She knelt in front of him and unzipped his pants.

With her delicate, well-manicured hand, she reached inside and pulled out a massive piece of meat. His dick was just like him, she thought—thick and husky, with a well-shaped head and silky hair. An erection was well under way.

She rubbed his pole between her palms, spat on the head, and began to lube the shaft. Then she placed her full red lips around the head and slid them down over the rim. She tapped his dickslit with the tip of her tongue, and gently nursed the dab of precome already forming there.

"Aw, man!" he grabbed her head and thrust his hips forward, forcing her to take his shaft all the way into her throat.

Sue had come home to relax, but relaxing her throat was even better! She took him in, and took him down, gobbling him up with a dinnertime hunger. All thoughts of her pizza had faded in light of this wholesome Italian sausage.

"Get up!" Suddenly the delivery boy sounded a bit less boyish.

She stopped her feasting and stood up in front of him. He reached out and tore her blouse open. Without warning, he twisted and pulled her hard nipples, making her wince. He leaned down and bit her nipple gently and then sucked as much as he could of her tit into his mouth. Apparently, he was just as hungry as she was!

Sue wanted more from her pizza man, and he wasn't about to disappoint her. With strength born of twenty-five deliveries a day, he picked her up and positioned her on the dining-room table. He lifted her skirt up, tore off her lace panties, and located her burning pussy. With his thumb, he stroked it several times and then inserted two fingers into her sopping-wet cunt. She spread her legs wide instinctively and lifted them over his shoulders for support. He was going to feed her his salami, and she was going to love it.

He propped himself on the table and, with dick in hand, he whacked her pussy repeatedly, making her sigh with ecstasy. She could feel the fire from the tips of her toes to the top of her head. She wanted nothing more than to be ravaged by his immense pole.

He guided his cock into her juicy cunt and pushed it in slowly, knowing from the way it felt that she never had anything so big and wide in her life. When it was all the way in, he held it in position, offering her a broad grin and gazing at her through heavy-lidded eyes. He reached down and kissed her, and he felt her body relax under his.

Then he started to pump her hard and fast. She cried out, shaking her head and lifting her hips to maximize the impact. He was relentless, locking her in a fierce gaze, and reaching in to pinch one of her nipples.

Sue steadied herself on her elbows and began to lick and nibble on his torso. She wanted to devour her pizza boy. He grabbed the hair behind her head and pulled it tight, restricting her, and started biting her neck.

That did it! Waves of immense, all-consuming pleasure washed up and down her body. This delivery boy was eating her and impaling her at the same time. She was coming!

He let her lie on the table motionless holding down her wrists over her head and he fucked her viciously. He licked the sweat that was trickling down her forehead. Suddenly, his whole body tensed. He stopped his pumping, held tightly onto her wrists, and with a deep, long breath, he shoved his cock as far in as it would go...and spilled his come.

He gave her a few more strokes before he pulled out. Sue sat up quickly and took his tool into her mouth, sucking out any sperm that may have been left behind.

They lay on the table for a little while, trying to catch their breath.

"I think the pizza is cold," Sue said.

"Don't worry. I'll give you a refund."

"Do you deliver on weekends?"

"I deliver seven days a week."

"Well, in that case, I may just be ordering seven days a week. And don't expect me to have small bills lying around!"

THE UNDERGROUND CLUB
Pat Loughton

I felt Mike's hands come up from behind me, cupping my breasts and squeezing them. He rubbed his bulge against my ass. He sat on the bench in our little cubicle, and I sat on his lap. He pulled my black slip-dress over my head, exposing my naked body. I leaned back on him and spread my legs and he started to play with my clit. We were both staring at the couple, fisting in the opposite cubicle. My nipples were aching with excitement.

This was our first visit to New York City, and we'd decided to explore the wild sex clubs we'd heard so much about. Mike is something of a voyeur, and a frequent visitor to the sex shops in our city. We're both very open-minded, and we enjoy sharing all kinds of sexual experiences with each other.

We'd picked up a local porn magazine and searched through the listings for a sex club. Back home, we were lucky if one existed within a hundred-mile radius. There were so many in New York, we almost lost count! I wet my panties just reading the ads!

A lean, swarthy man passed by our cubicle and looked in. He stopped by the corner of the door, pulled out his cock, and started stroking it. That really sent me over the edge. I wanted to get fucked right there in public, for everyone to see. I started tweaking my nipples, staring him in the eyes. He licked his lips and stroked faster. He was being respectful of our space.

"Do you want him?" Mike whispered in my ear.

"Yes, I do," I replied loud enough for the man to hear me.

"Come on in," Mike told the man.

The man kneeled in front of me and kissed my hand. He thanked Mike and me for letting him join us. I took both his hands and placed them on my breasts. He began to squeeze them gently, pinching my hardened nipples, and tugging at them lightly. My pussy was dripping. Mike was fingering my hole and licking my neck.

"I wan fuck you," Mike said.

He lifted my hips, pulled out his dick, and had me sit down on it. Mike sighed with pleasure. Our anonymous friend was still sucking on me while stroking his own cock hard and fast. The doorway behind him was becoming crowded with men, pulling on their cocks and staring at the three of us.

"Lick my clit!" I told my new friend.

He reached down between my legs and pulled my

pussylips apart. He had a fast tongue. He licked with fervor as I humped Mike with a slow, languorous rhythm. I stared up at the crowd of jerkers and plucked at my nipples, smiling at them. I heard them moan, some louder than others. Some were jostling in from behind, but not one of them passed the barrier of the door.

Mike pushed me up, pulling off his T-shirt, and stood behind me. Bending me over, he inserted his cock inside my tight asshole, making me cry out against the feeling of the pleasure and pain together. Pumping me from behind, he pulled my head up to face our horny guest.

"Suck it!" Mike ordered me.

I took the man's cock and greedily shoved it in my mouth. I slurped sloppily on it, like one of those Italian ices we'd picked up in the Village. I rocked my head back and forth and sucked hard, occasionally letting it drop out of my mouth and watching it bob back up in front of my lips. It only made him jerk off faster!

I rode Mike's throbbing meat without mercy, slapping my bottom against him as I pumped my hips back and forth. I wanted his cock pushed through me. I was still pumping frantically when Mike shot his load of hot come into me. I continued to pump even after he pulled out. I was burning hot.

Mike pulled his dick out and wiped it on the crack of my ass. He then massaged his sticky load all around my asscheeks and then slid his fingers between my legs, teasing my clit with his middle finger, until I had fire shooting up the insides of my thighs. He stuck three fingers in my cunt and pumped me hard and fast. I shuddered uncontrollably and came violently a second time—still holding the stranger's cock in my mouth.

I grabbed his ass and pushed my face onto his massive meat. I reached behind and worked my finger into the ass of my standing lover, wriggling it inside his tight hole. I could feel his cock flex in my mouth, and set to sucking him as hard as I could. His cock went rigid inside my mouth, his balls pulled tight, and his asscheeks gripped my finger. I pulled him out of my mouth quickly and pulled at his cock just a few more times before he shot his load all over my sweaty tits. He reached out and rubbed his goo all over my breasts pushing his hot palms against my bullet-hard nipples.

"Thank you, my lady."

"My pleasure," I replied.

"And thank you, sir, for allowing me to join you," he said to Mike.

Mike smiled at him and looked at me. He pulled me into his arms and gave me a passionate kiss. "Anything for my baby."

We looked up only to see the half a dozen men of all shapes and sizes shooting their loads by the doorway! We picked up our clothes and squeezed through the crowd. I must admit, I did grab a cock or two as I made my way out of there!

FOREVER FRIENDS
Guy Jeremy

A few months back, I got together with my college buddy Steve, whom I hadn't seen in over five years. Since then he had married a gorgeous gal, and he made it clear that he was just dying for me to meet her.

Cathy was as pretty as Steve had described her, and had a sweet personality to match. She took a liking to me right away, and our first evening together was a hit. They invited me back for the following week, and I accepted gladly. I really wanted Steve to be part of my life once again. We really had some good times, way back when.

I showed up for our second dinner date with a bouquet of flowers for Cathy and a bottle of Jack Daniel's for Steve. It was the least I could do to show my appreciation for the two of them. They were both very happy to see me and we immediately slid back into some great food and deep conversation. Afterward, we sat around the fireplace, talking about ex-girlfriends and some of our raunchier escapades. Cathy seemed genuinely interested, and I was surprised at her willingness to talk about some of her own. She was one sexy woman!

When Cathy went to get us some more Jack Daniel's, Steve mentioned how much she liked me, and how she wanted to get to know me a lot better. I was a little confused, but he told me that she found me attractive and, wildest of all, that they were interested in experimenting with a third person.

I couldn't believe my ears! Cathy walked back into the room with a tray of drinks. Realizing quickly what the conversation was about, she joined in.

Of course I had no objection to this, but I was a little concerned about handling the situation. Cathy put her hand on mine and told me that she had heard so many nice things about me from Steve, it made sense that they would approach the only person who they felt could be trusted and was fun-loving at the same time. So I decided to relax and let them lead the way.

Cathy dimmed the lights and lit some scented candles. Steve and I sat next to each other on the sofa. I still felt a little awkward. Cathy came over to me, sat on my lap, and gave me a shot of bourbon. She thanked me for being a sport about this and kissed me on the cheek. She then unbuttoned the front of her dress and exposed her small, firm breasts. Clearly taking charge, she took my hand and asked me to feel them.

Her breasts were perfect, with just the right amount of firmness and bounce. I could feel my dick harden, and I kept trying to fight the urge to glance up at Steve. God, were those tits gorgeous! I leaned over and began to suck on Cathy's eraserlike nipples.

After a while, she stood up and took off her dress. Steve had pulled his cock out and was stroking it aggressively. He had an enormous hard-on. Cathy stripped completely, lay down on the soft rug directly in front of us, and began to play with herself sensually. My heart was beating so fast, I thought it would burst. I pulled out my cock and began stroking it, forcing myself to lock eyes with Cathy, watching her lick her lips.

The three of us were masturbating simultaneously, watching each other and enjoying every minute of it. Cathy changed poses a few more times, showing off that hot body to its best effect in the firelight. Sweeping her legs gracefully over her head, she gave us a clear view of her smooth, toned ass, and I thrilled to the pucker of her snatch. She fingered her asshole while playing with her pussy, making me want her so badly.

Steve moved beside her and motioned for me to join him. In seconds she was sliding one cock in each hand, pumping us to fever pitch before sucking on us in turn.

Steve and I pinched and pulled on her nipples while she gave us head. I reached down and slowly, cautiously, starting fingering her pussy. She let out a long, sweet sigh in response. Her cunt was soaking wet.

Steve winked at me. In that instant, I knew it would be okay to fuck his wife. I nodded and smiled at him

before positioning myself between her long legs. Taking hold of my swollen dick, I probed her, feeling her soaking, fiery pussy stretch as I thrust.

I looked up to see Steve fucking her face. What a sight! Her face wasn't even visible! She was just a body being fucked from both ends. She massaged Steve's balls and fingered his asshole while he was dick-feeding her. I leaned in and helped myself to her lovely nipples. The pleasure we were giving her was making her gasp for air, and I heard her muffled moans.

I sucked her nipples hard, biting them occasionally. I increased my pumping motions and pushed my cock harder and harder into that fantastic snatch. I could feel her body tense under mine. Suddenly she began to cry out and tremble. I felt her hot pussy contract violently. I knew she was coming!

I fucked her like a savage. I sucked, bit and chewed on her breasts until I couldn't bear it any longer. Her pussy contractions were so intense, my dick felt like it was being drawn right into her body, forced to become a part of her being. My balls tightened. My heart was racing. Finally I exploded like a cannon into her tight cunt, filling her with my come.

My head spinning, I looked up to see Steve stroking his massive shaft furiously, while Cathy was sucking on his balls and fingering his asshole. Panting now, he gave his dick a couple of final strokes and stuffed it quickly between her lips. He shot his load into her mouth, filling it until his come oozed out of the corners.

The three of us were exhausted, but Steve and Cathy

were all smiles. They thanked me for being so great about this and asked me if I was interested in having regular sessions with them. It didn't take too much thought for me to tell them to count me in! I also told them that one day, when I had a girl all my own, they had to promise to let her become a part of our little group as well. The two of them were struck by the thought, realizing the endless possibilities, and told me that this looked like the rekindling of a beautiful friendship!

BOTTOMS UP
Stewart Oldson

Don pulled out his massive erection and brandished it at Sandy like a double-barreled shotgun. It was thick and long, ridged with veins, capped with a fat purple head. He was sitting on the large leather sofa with his legs spread apart, staring at the girl kneeling in front of him, making sure she knew he meant business.

Sandy was petite, with short platinum-blonde hair, large brown eyes, small tits, and a huge, voluptuous ass. Her hairy pussy had full pink lips and had been trimmed neatly for the occasion. She had been mesmerized by Don's stare, awaiting his next set of instructions eagerly. Her pussy was dripping wet from excitement, waiting for his fat pole to fill her up.

"Come here, bitch!" he ordered. "Put your hands

behind your back and suck my cock, slow and sloppy, until I tell you to stop."

Sandy moved closer to him, opened her hungry mouth and lowered her head over his massive penis. She swallowed it all the way down to his balls, then slowly pulled up, leaving a glistening trail of saliva on his shaft. She closed her lips around his head and circled her tongue around the rim a couple of times. Then she sucked his head slow and hard before swallowing his shaft a second time. She wanted to touch his cock and balls so badly, but she had to keep her hands behind her back.

"Faster!" he commanded.

She listened to him, her head bobbing faster, even as his dick grew thicker. He could hear her slurping at his pole as if it were an ice-cream cone in a Texas August. Her spit was dripping slowly down to his balls.

"Enough!" Don yanked her face away, and roughly tossed her onto her back. He had almost come. "Turn around, lean forward, and spread your legs!"

Without a word, she obliged. He spread her asscheeks, spat in his palm, and wiped the makeshift lube on her pink little asshole. He licked two of his fingers and slowly probed her tight hole. She drew a quick breath and let out a low moan, surprised that he went for her ass. She'd thought for sure she'd be pussy-fucked by him. This was even better!

Sandy lowered her head and torso all the way to the floor, arched her back, and pushed her ass as far up as she could. Don started moving his fingers in and out in a slow rhythmic motion. He even deigned to lean down and spit into the action before inserting a third finger. This time a louder moan escaped Sandy's lips, and she opened her legs a little wider.

"You're ready for me, cunt!"

Pulling out his digits, he stroked his dick a few times, and headed into her primed sphincter. He inserted the head, but then pulled it out, teasing her, forcing her to whimper with fear and anticipation. This time, he put the head in again, and held it there, a certain warning of things to come!

He started to slap her fat, meaty ass and enjoyed watching it jiggle. Then, without mercy, he rammed the rest of his cock all the way in and fucked her with a couple of fast, hard strokes. Sandy was gasping.

"Shut your mouth and take it!" he ordered sternly.

Sandy was worried that she wouldn't be able to stay quiet. Don grabbed her hips and started butt-slamming her rapidly and viciously. Sandy's breathing accelerated. She was biting down on her lips in a desperate effort not to make a sound. Tightening his hold, Don increased his force, fucking her ass until his balls smacked her pussylips, making her clit throb. She reached between her legs and tweaked her love-button, sending flames of ecstasy shooting through her body.

Don's cock and balls stiffened. With a couple of strokes, he shot his wad violently into her anus. He knew she had come, and like the good girl that she was, she had not made a peep.

"Clean it!"

Sandy turned around quickly and took his dick in her mouth. She sucked all the remaining come out of his hole and then swallowed his shaft one last time. When all the goo was gone from his cock, she worked on his balls with hungry kitten licks until they, too, were spotless. When she was done, she looked up at him with a big smile.

"Good girl." He cupped her face with his palms, leaned down, and gave her a long kiss. "Now go get me a beer."

FRAT BOYS

Laura Mallory

My new sorority girlfriends told me that if I was to make it through initiation, I had to please a select group of young gentlemen from the best fraternity on campus. Three seniors had been chosen specifically for me, and I was instructed to please them in every way. I would be their property for one whole night. It was either that, or no sisterhood, and eternal damnation for the next four years!

I wore a powder-blue satin mini-dress, silver strap sandals, and a garter belt with white silk stockings. I have to admit that I was a little nervous, but I'd never been with more than one man at a time, and the thought of doing something like this had grown too exciting to resist.

A tall blond man opened the door and introduced himself as Chuck. I told him my name was Samantha, and he let me in with a flourish. It seemed that they had the whole place to themselves. He introduced me to Jim and Andrew, and to my delight, they were all very handsome athletic types.

Andrew got me a drink and the other two served themselves. We chatted for a while until we felt comfortable with each other, and Andrew made sure that my glass was always full. They seemed to be treating me with a certain degree of respect, and I liked that.

"My sisters made some good choices in you guys. I must say, they have very good taste." I told them with a smile. "I knew I could trust them."

"The girls are extremely thoughtful, and we aim to please!" Jim smiled. "We've been exchanging freshmen for years, and it almost always works out. When our freshman brothers pledge our fraternity, the last step in their initiation is to get a thorough training session led by your sorority sisters. We were all trained by them, and when you pass your initiation, you'll be in a position to train our new guys."

I hadn't really heard all the details of this agreement before, but I thought it was a great idea. I couldn't wait to get my first freshman brother to train. This was extra motivation for me to please the boys as much as I could!

"Why don't we get started?"

"By all means, Samantha!" Chuck said with a big bright smile.

I got up in front of the three of them, slipped out of

my satin dress, and threw it at Andrew, who folded it neatly and put it aside. They were all fixated on my breasts. I smiled and pinched my nipples to harden them. Teasingly, I removed my panties, but I kept my stockings on and my high-heeled sandals. I squatted and began to stroke my pussy with one hand while playing with my nipples with the other.

The boys were all warm and toasty now, and I could see the huge bulges in their pants. I knew they were getting pretty uncomfortable.

"Now it's your turn to strip for me!" I told them.

In seconds they were on their feet, and clothes were flying everywhere. The three of them had immense cocks. Andrew was the only one who wasn't cut. They stood in front of me, like a sexy police lineup, their stiff poles bobbing and pointing at me.

I strutted toward them, and kneeled down and gave each dick a quick lick. The three of them shuddered in unison. It was such a great sight! I took turns sucking each dick and each set of balls until the three of them were sufficiently lubed with my saliva. My body was burning with anticipation. I wanted more than anything to get fucked by all of them at the same time.

"Jim, I want to sit on your dick, I want Chuck to fuck my ass, and I want to suck your beautiful uncut dick, Andrew!"

"Man! She's taken control of the situation!" Jim laughed. "I guess we'll make an exception in your case, Sam!"

They looked at each other and with a smile and a nod

they immediately positioned themselves on the plush carpeted floor. Jim immediately struck the best pose, lying down, all hunky and muscular, looking up at me. I straddled him and guided his monstrous rod into my soaking-wet pussy.

I could feel my lips spread as the head of his cock pushed its way in, stretching me wide. I breathed deeply, shifted my thighs, and finally he was all the way in. I leaned forward and asked him to suck on my nipples. He did so gladly.

Chuck moved in behind me. He pulled my asscheeks apart, licked two of his fingers, inserted them into my tight asshole, and fingered me slowly in preparation for his cock. After he worked it for a while, he pulled his fingers out and replaced them with the head of his cock. He pushed in slowly, and I felt my hole stretch like it had never done before. I have to admit that I was no virgin, but no one had fucked my ass until that night. It was pretty painful, but I breathed deeply and slowly to relax myself.

Chuck continued to push stretching my hole farther and farther. Finally it was all the way in. Once my asshole adjusted, the pain turned into unbelievable pleasure.

My pussy and asshole were plugged by two enormous cocks; before long, each was pumping away. I was delirious with ecstasy. I'd never known how much pleasure one person could experience. I felt insatiable and I wanted more.

Andrew was standing in front of me stroking his shaft. I grabbed his dick and pushed back the foreskin, exposing a fat knob of a head that twinkled with precome. This was the icing on the cake. I shoved his meat in my mouth and sucked it wildly. I was being fucked in every orifice, and I loved every minute of it. I only wished I had two more dicks to stroke!

Chuck was pumping my ass, I was pumping Jim's dick, and Andrew was fucking my face. All I could hear were moans, flesh pounding flesh, and heavy breathing. The four of us were fucking in rhythmic motions, as if we'd been rehearsing this for a play in the theater club!

Chuck increased his speed, and I thought my asshole would get torn apart. The combination of pleasure and pain made me dizzy. He fucked my ass with such vigor that his balls slapped my bottom. Jim was thrusting his hips with such force that Andrew's cock had nowhere to go but way down my open throat. Andrew held my head, his knees slightly bent, and he fucked my face with a football jock's cheerful sense of abandon.

I couldn't hold out any more. My pussyjuices were all over Jim's dick. His balls were completely soaked. I held unto Andrew's buttocks firmly and, with a sudden burst, I climaxed violently. Andrew's thick meat muffled my screams, but Chuck and Jim felt my contractions.

Chuck shoved his dick as far into my hole as it would go—and exploded. He thrust a few times, emptying himself completely inside my sore ass. He pulled out quickly and surprised me by licking his come from my hole. I could tell that Jim was ready to burst because I felt his body tense under me. He pushed up, lifting me slightly off the floor, groaning like a hungry pig—and with one final thrust, he shot his load deep into my cunt. I squeezed my pussy muscles tightening around his dick, which made him moan even more loudly.

Andrew was in his own little world, fucking my mouth. I massaged his balls with one hand. With my other, I searched for his asshole. Once I found it, I inserted my index finger and twirled it around. This was too much for Andrew. I felt his balls tighten. His asshole squeezed shut. Then, with a sudden shove, he fired into my mouth like a machine gun, drowning me with his hot, creamy liquid. I swallowed as much as I could, and continued to suck him until his dick dropped from exhaustion in my mouth. I had sucked him dry.

The three of us lay on the floor, smoking and sipping some wine. According to my sorority sisters, I had to keep this up all night! Andrew got up and poured me another drink.

"I can't remember ever feeling so good," I confessed.

"You know, I think you're already qualified to train our freshmen brothers, Samantha." Chuck smiled. "But let's follow the rules anyway, shall we?"

"Here, here!" Jim chimed in, and we raised our glasses to the toast.

I'll never forget that night. I'm now the top trainer for the fraternity; and, if I do say so myself, they've all turned out to be the finest!

THE VIRGIN
Timothy Host

Judy had long, straight dark brown hair and pale skin, beautiful soft tits, and a slender body. She had never been with a man before, and she was frightened at what might happen. I had some concerns myself since, admittedly, I'd never been with a virgin before. I was concerned about hurting her, but the idea was way too exciting for me to worry too much.

Though she had just graduated from high school, Judy had managed to stay a virgin, which is somewhat shocking nowadays, I suppose. We'd met at a friend's party last winter and had been dating on and off for months. Sometimes I had to bite my tongue to keep from pushing her. But tonight, with its cool summer breeze and strawberry wine, seemed to be just the right time for her to give up her cherry. So she asked me to make love to her.

She was lying naked under the covers, watching my every move. I dimmed the lights, shucked off my clothes, and joined her in bed. I rubbed up against her soft body and kissed her face, her neck, her breasts. She put her arms around me and gave me a gentle kiss. Her nipples were hard and I touched them, licking them and brushing my fingertips against them until she started to sigh.

I reached down between her legs, spread her pussylips, and started massaging her clit gently. Her back arched pushing her torso against mine. I continued to rub her virgin pussy until I felt wetness coat my fingers. She was ready for me.

I pushed her legs farther apart and got on top of her. I rubbed my erection up and down her dewy love-mound, getting her more aroused with every move. This was usually as far as we got—a nice wet-hump and nothing more. But tonight I was going to deflower my pretty Judy, and nothing was going to stop us.

Her hands were around my neck, stroking my hair and my ears occasionally. We continued to kiss passionately, nibbling on each other's lips, exploring each other's mouths, teeth, faces. She smelled like roses, and her hair was silky soft. She particularly liked it when I licked her hard nipples and suckled them gently.

She wrapped her legs around mine and moved her hips to the rhythm of my circular motions. I knew she was ready for more. My hard-on poked and pushed until it found her little virgin hole.

"I want you to guide it in," I whispered.

She sighed and nodded. I could tell she was nervous. She was about to push something huge into the tiny hole between her legs. But she also seemed determined, and I loved her for it.

I rested my thick cockhead on her opening, and firmly but gently, I entered her. She was incredibly tight. Her body tensed and she moaned loudly. I could tell it was a mix of pleasure and pain. I felt her pussy open slowly around my thick, fat meat.

I pushed all the way in and held it there for a moment, kissing her and sucking in her essence. She gasped—and I could swear I heard an audible pop. She was all mine!

I shoved my dick deep into her and then I began pumping her slow and hard, forcing her to get used to my manhood. I held her wrists down, stared her straight in the eyes, and continued to fuck her, now increasing my speed. I was going to break her in real good.

She was mesmerized by my gaze. She looked confused and pleased at the same time. She was under my control, and she would stay pinned under me until I was done. I pulled my cock out and shoved it back in, stretching her all over again. I did this a few times, teasing her with my meat until she was moaning nonstop. I decided to get rougher with her nipples, so I started biting them and pinching them.

She was thrusting her hips up at me faster and faster, now, responding to me by indulging herself. She whimpered and moaned, and shook her head from side to side as her body shook beneath me. Her pussy was so tight that her contractions made my dick feel as if it was being pulled inside her, grabbed and sucked into my virgin baby. I opened her legs wider than they already had been, lifted them over her shoulders, and fucked her fast and furious, my balls slapping her ass. I continued until I exploded, filling her up with loads of come for the very first time. I pulled my dick out and forced her to take it in the mouth. She sucked me clean and swallowed every bit of come that was left. I kissed her to show my appreciation.

Judy must have been very satisfied because we've been fucking every day since then. Her pussy is still very tight, but my dick slides in with just a little more ease. On the other hand, she still has a virgin ass. I think I'll be stretching that out just a bit pretty soon, as well!

WORKPLACE SCANDAL

Linda Garcia

Mr. Marco looked busy as usual when Sissy stepped into his office, pad and pen in hand. She wore a skintight blue business suit, high-heeled shoes, and a shiny gold chain around her neck. Spicy perfume filled the room, making her boss take notice of her stunning presence.

She sat in the leather chair across from him, crossed her long legs, and rested her pad on her knee, ready to take notes. At this point, Mr. Marco forgot why he'd called her in. He was clearly focused on her legs.

"Are you okay, Mr. Marco?"

"I'm just fine, Sissy."

"Would you like for me to get you a cup of coffee?"

"No, that's all right," he laughed. "You just happen to look especially beautiful today, and it's hard for me to concentrate."

Sissy was amused by his remark. She'd been hot for her boss from the day she started at the firm, but he'd always seemed to be cool toward her. Apparently an opportunity was presenting itself!

"Why, thank you, Mr. Marco." She recrossed her legs. "That's quite a compliment. How would you like to see some more of me?"

"What do you mean, Sissy?"

"Oh, Mr. Marco! I know you're not as naïve as you'd have me think."

She stood up and unbuttoned her jacket exposing her large breasts. She unzipped her skirt and let it drop to the floor. Stepping over her skirt, she walked over to his desk and leaned over. "You've seen what I look like. Would you like to have a taste?"

He rose to his feet immediately and walked around his desk. He unhooked her black lace bra and cupped her breasts. Her pink nipples were long and hard. He pushed her tits together and sucked both nipples into his mouth. He suckled them until they turned bright red.

Sissy leaned backward onto the desk, making it convenient for her boss to pull down her silk stockings and black lace panties. Maneuvering between her legs, he dove into her rosy pussy, first nibbling on her plump labia, then flicking her clit with the tip of his tongue. Sissy trembled at his touch and spread her legs wider.

Mr. Marco unzipped his fly and unleashed his giant erection. It was dripping with precome. Holding it in position, he led it straight into her hungry cunt. Sissy leaned back on her elbows and slid her legs over his shoulders for support. At long last, her boss would be hers!

Holding firmly onto her thighs, he pumped Sissy at a leisurely pace, enjoying the feel of her tight, wet pussy. He fucked his secretary as he watched her play with her sensitive nipples, then grabbed for her tits and massaged them roughly. The intense sensations made Sissy want to scream, but, discretion being the better part of valor, she held back.

She leaned back and purred as he continued his onslaught, filling her up with his bloated cock for the very first time. She reached down between her legs and rubbed her clit vigorously, keeping it up until her body convulsed and she came with a furor.

He pulled out his dick and rubbed it on her soaking-wet pussy. He lifted her legs over her head and plunged his swollen cock into her tight asshole. She took a deep breath, feeling the pain as he stretched her sphincter to new limits.

With a few strokes, he felt an intense heaviness from the depths of his balls. His scrotum tensed as the sensation traveled up his shaft through to the tip of his cockhead and exploded his steamy come inside Sissy's stretched out asshole. He kept his cock inside her until he was completely drained and then pulled out, rubbing his cock up and down her crack.

Mr. Marco sat on the leather chair he had purchased especially for his secretary, then took a few deep breaths. Sissy got up and walked over to him, picking up her pad and pen.

"Mr. Marco, now that your head has been cleared, do you remember what you had called me in for?"

"Yes." He cleared his throat and looked up at Sissy with a sly smile. "I wanted you to take some notes on employer/employee relations. But I think there are going to be some last-minute adjustments."

ROADHOG
Sam Spears

Spike grabbed Ellen's T-shirt and ripped it off her body. She gasped, but she wasn't afraid of him. He ran a finger along her large, succulent breasts, passing it over her thick, erect nipples, and circled them. She shivered. Spike's cock pushed against the worn-out denim of his jeans.

Ellen was barely legal, but "very mature for her age." And she knew what pleased her. She'd been after Spike for some time, but he'd been playing it cool and ignored her until her most recent birthday. Now he had every intention of teaching her how he liked things done.

Spike put his huge hand around her long, silky throat, his fingers meeting at the nape of her neck. He brought his mouth down onto hers and licked her full, hungry lips. His free hand roamed her body, feeling her ribs, rubbing her soft belly and sliding down her pants.

He wanted to ram the hard-on in his jeans right up her fresh young ass. He moved in on her, pressing her frail body against the wall with his. As if it had a mind of its own, his cock struggled to get free. Keeping a secure hold around her throat, he finally unzipped his fly and stroked his aching rod.

"Take 'em off, cunt," he hissed in her face.

She kicked out of her pants and panties while he stroked his shaft, preparing it for her tender ass. He nearly came when he saw her naked body, soft and smooth with a clean shaven cunt. His huge hunk of prime beef stood at attention, also awaiting its master's next order. Ellen reached out to touch it. Her fingers were cool and soft against his flesh.

"I didn't give you permission to do that!" he breathed.

She pulled her hand away immediately. Spike looked her up and down, examining her nakedness. Ellen felt self-conscious and vulnerable. She wasn't used to being ogled out in the open with no clothes on. He turned her around and pressed her face up against the wall. She grunted at the force he used.

Spike spread her asscheeks and inserted a finger into her tight little hole without bothering to prime the way. He pushed in and out, and then inserted a second. Her hole was hot and moist, grabbing his finger as if he'd placed it in a baby's palm. She was breathing heavily, leaning her forehead up against the brick wall.

Spike removed his fingers and lubed his massive cock with his spit. Pressing her neck to hold her securely, he took her hard from behind and rammed his huge cock up her tight little ass. She was so aroused, she hardly even cried out as she felt him entering. Spike plunged into her roughly, stretching her virgin asshole to the max. He didn't even seem to care that her face kept thumping softly against the wall every time she was prodded. He was a ravenous animal, pouncing on his tender young prey. This was the price she paid for straying too close!

Her tits were slapping against the wall when Spike raised a hand to feel them up. He pinched her nipples hard, pleased with her grunts and moans of pleasure. With his free hand, Spike reached around her front and rubbed her clit, hard and strong, making it throb. She came screaming, her body twisting and turning, her pussyjuices streaming down her thighs.

That did it for Spike. He exploded inside of her, torrents of hot come firing inside her ravaged shithole. It backed up as he pulled out, leaking down the back of her thighs and dripping off his dick. She turned quickly, then knelt and sucked the come from his cock, making sure it was cleaned and shiny after all that hard, dirty work.

He leaned back against his motorcycle and took a few deep breaths. Ellen seemed to be more than gratified. Dutifully so.

"That's good, cunt." Spike stroked her hair. "Now you know what to expect from me. I need to be able to fuck you any way and any time I like. That's just the way things've got to be. Being on the road like we will, you've got to take what you can get, when you can get it. Tomorrow we can be just a smear on the asphalt, y'know?"

Ellen nodded. She wanted that lifestyle, and she was willing to sacrifice anything for this kind of lay. Hot, sleazy sex, a fast bike, and a rough man…

"What more can I ask for?" She grinned.

A LEAGUE OF HER OWN

Fred Richards

Katy was the neighborhood tomboy. She didn't care what anyone thought about the way she looked or dressed, or how she liked to play rough with the boys. She was always involved in some tough sport, giving and getting a pounding, not worried about the bumps and bruises she'd accumulated over the years.

Now she found herself pinned down by Ron the quarterback, the victim of one of his patented tackles. He was the biggest, toughest guy on the block, and Katy was just a plaything to him. Today, probably because his teammates were studying back in the dorms, he humored her need to be one of the guys. She had more than the slightest idea that he secretly lusted after her, but that was only something she'd hidden. It was the thrill of the chase that she enjoyed—especially if the chase involved a pigskin and some warm green grass.

She was struggling to get loose, but Ron's weight and strength made it more than hopeless. He held her by the wrists and without warning he reached down and stuck his tongue down into her mouth. Katy bit him and turned her head quickly in disgust.

"Ow! What's the matter with you?" he shouted, looking like a little boy who had skinned his knee. "Are you a dyke or something?"

"I'm no dyke!" she hissed at him, confused at what had just happened.

"I like you, Katy. I didn't mean to scare you," his voice softened.

Katy's body relaxed and she smiled at him. She kind of liked being pinned down by a big muscular guy. Maybe that's why she enjoyed playing with them so much. She liked the roughness as much as she liked the game.

She picked her head up and kissed Ron back. This time, it was *her* tongue doing the deep dive into *his* mouth. Ron made an agreeable noise and hummed into her, kissing her back noisily.

He let go of her wrists and Katy pulled her shirt off. Her tits were the size of baseballs, with little hard red nipples. He grabbed a hold of them and stuffed them one by one into his mouth taking turns sucking on them. He nibbled and bit her nipples gently, sending waves of pleasure throughout her body.

She stood up and looked around. As she suspected,

the park was empty. Finals had a tendency to clear the place. She removed her shorts and panties. Ron watched her as he freed his own meat from his jockstrap. His cock was thick and smooth, like a streamlined rocket, except that it curved slightly to the left. Katy giggled at it, but her eyes betrayed some true lust. She sat in front of him spread her legs and slowly rubbed her clit. Ron kneeled in front of her, pushed her legs further apart, and guided his manhood into her tender pink pussy.

He entered her slowly, feeling her pussy muscles stretch. She moaned and thrust her hips forward to take him in. His cock was being swallowed by her hot, juicy cunt. Once he was all the way in, he began to pump her hard and fast. He kissed her neck, her face, and her ears, making her grunt and shake from the sensations. This game was still relatively new to her; but as with every other sport, she was a natural.

Katy played with her nipples, getting off on Ron watching her enjoy herself. The pounding of his huge cock was making her feel better and better, but she retained control and continued teasing him with her little show.

Ron slowed down and flipped Katy onto her side. Now in the spoon position, he continued to prod her without skipping a beat. He found her clit and stroked it, slowly at first, then increasing the speed until she couldn't bear it any longer. With a loud scream, her body jerked and twisted until she climaxed.

Katy's pussy was contracting now, giving Ron's cock the sensation of being squeezed and sucked at the same time. The contractions made her cunt feel even tighter than it had been. Ron increased his pace and fucked her harder. His ballsac tightened and he finally shot a hot, steamy load of thick come inside her throbbing cunt. He pumped a few more times, making sure he was completely drained before pulling out and rolling over on the grass.

Katy was ready for more, but she realized that Ron needed some time to rest. She started playing with her pussy and licking her fingers as the football stud looked on, pleased at the sight. He reached for her tits and, massaged them gently. He liked scoring high at his games, and this was no exception. He'd spent long months building his stamina, and he intended to stick to the playbook as long as she would have him. Together they would certainly make a winning team!

ROCK 'N' ROLL
Art Collins

The guys were wrapping up their rehearsal session when Jenny walked in. The no-nonsense studio manager was there to collect the money they owed for the recording time. Gary pulled out a wad of bills and handed it to her.

"Hey, aren't you gonna play that tape for me?" she asked. "I'd like to hear your latest pieces."

Gary was thrilled at her interest and told the guys to take off without him.

"I didn't think you'd be interested in this kinda music, Jen." He popped in the tape and turned up the volume.

"I guess I'm full of surprises," she answered, eyeing his ass as he toyed with the knobs.

Though she rarely let on, Jenny liked the blaring heavy-metal band. And though Gary's band tended toward the mediocre, Gary himself did not. She'd been turned on by the way he played his bass guitar. Any man who could strum those heavy strings with such a stunning tempo had to be good for one or two more things in life!

Gary could see her nipples hardening as the beat got more intense. He leaned over and unbuttoned her blouse; and she sat back, letting him take control. Her breasts were perfectly round and large, with huge dark nipples. He passed his fingers over them, making her shudder. She lifted up her skirt and showed Gary her dripping pussy. She never wore panties. She liked feeling free.

Gary slipped a pair of fingers into her soaking cunt and pushed hard, flicking her clit with his thumb. She moaned and squirmed in her chair, begging him for more. He stood up and unzipped his pants, releasing his tremendous erect cock. It seemed disproportionate to his tall, skinny frame.

He shoved his pole into her hungry pussy, and it slid right in. He fucked to the beat of his music, thrusting hard and fast. She tilted her head back and screamed, her voice blending in with the blare and garbled lyrics of the song. He slapped her breasts and tugged on her nipples. Jenny liked to have her tits treated roughly. She held her breasts steady for him, and he gripped them hard as he pounded her pussy.

The intense pleasure made Jenny dizzy. She came so hard, she almost fell off the couch. Gary held her down and rammed her until he, too, was ready to come.

Before very long, he pulled out his cock and shoved it

into her mouth. He fucked her face for half a track more. Then he exploded during his bass solo, shooting his load into her throat. She gulped it down, finally satisfying her hunger for Gary's rock-'n'-roll dick.

Gary pulled his cock out of her mouth and got dressed. Jenny sat naked in her chair, watching his every move. He was good, she thought to herself; but for their next session, she was going to give the drummer a chance, then the lead guitar, and when she had done them all, she'd have the band all at once. Yes, she was choosy. But sometimes she had to tell herself, what the hell! This was the best job she ever had!

ON THE BEAT
Bobby Drakes

Michelle was handcuffed to the headboard of the bed in the doggy position, stripped of all her clothing. She was waiting in silence as the officer removed his gear. He knelt behind her, admiring her fleshy heart-shaped ass. He wore only his shirt, unbuttoned to expose his muscular torso, and his shades. His gun was out of reach, but he'd held on to his nightstick.

He tapped the inside of her thighs. She knew instinctively what that meant and obeyed, spreading them wider. Gently, now, he tapped her pussy with the heavy wooden baton, sending tingling sensations across her naked body. She left streaks of pussyjuice on his nightstick.

His dick was standing at attention. It was large and thick with an enormous head. He was a stern man who took what he wanted and gave no explanations to anyone. He had been a cop for over a decade, and had disciplined many unruly women. None of them ever complained, though.

He'd caught Michelle jaywalking earlier that day and, quickly taking note of her interest, offered her an interesting choice. Blow a day paying a fine down at the county courthouse, or blow *him* this afternoon. She'd opted for the latter. Right now, she was well on her way to realizing she had made the right choice.

He inserted three fingers up her cunt and pushed deep inside. Her pussy was tight, but her increasing wetness made his fingers slide in without effort. He twisted his fingers around, feeling the membranes of her cunt stretch and retract around them. She grunted and lifted her ass up, granting him easy access.

He removed his fingers and replaced them with his nightstick. He pushed it in gently, until it was in as far as it would go. She was moaning loudly with her eyes closed, moving her hips from side to side. He let go of the stick and primed her asshole with his saliva. Then, without another moment's notice, he stuffed her hole with his enormous cock—pushing all the way, not at all concerned about any discomfort he might be causing.

Gasping, eyes bulging, doing whatever she could to ease her pain, she took him. Her tight asshole enveloped his meat pole, even as his nightstick dangled from her cunt. With one fast thrust, he was all the way in. She jumped and screamed, her tits bouncing, absorbing the shock. He grabbed the stick and pushed it in and out as he pumped her ass with his meat. He was working her hard now, stuffing her from both ends.

Michelle swiveled her hips, pushing back to meet his hard thrusts. She wanted to please him as much as he wanted to discipline her. He slapped her asscheeks over and over, leaving nasty red handprints. He was relentless with her. With each passing moment, her yelling got louder, until he ordered her to shut her mouth. She bit her lips in response, groaning quietly as he proceeded toward climax.

He pounded her harder and harder until she came. Her pussy was soaked, and his dick churned its juices into a buttery froth. He held her hips tightly and pushed and pulled violently, until, at long last, he shot a steamy wad of thick come into her ravaged asshole. He pulled out his cock and tapped it in her crack draining every last bit drop.

He got out of the bed, got dressed, and removed the handcuffs. She collapsed, trying to roll up into a ball on the bed, but he did not let her.

"I think you've learned your lesson for now." He stroked her hair. "But I'm going to be watching you. One wrong move—and you're fucked!"

WSP

Julian Anthony Guerra

I sit there that October afternoon and watch a show, until I turn around quickly to see who's tickling my back, where my leather jacket and T-shirt had hiked. I'd seen her around the park since last June. Smiled at her. But I never thought she'd nibble.

She was a fox, all fluffy-haired and black-mascaraed, her summer body poured into autumn jeans and cutaway thermals. She's looking the other way, as if she didn't do it, but there's no one else around.

I ask her, "Why'd you do that?"

She says, " 'Cause you were there." And then she grins.

I stand up to face her. She's making it no secret that she's checking me out up close. Fine. Buys me time to do the same.

Running my gaze over her ripe breasts, to the soft

crescent of belly peeping out from under her cutoff thermals, I tell her, "It's getting a little chilly out."

"You kidding?" she says, as she breathes in strong and stretches wide. "It feels great. Looks great, too. Do you lift?"

Her lip gloss looks delicious. "Yeah, when I can."

She reaches in my jacket and feels a pec, then takes a few quick pokes around my gut. Then she slides a finger lower and pushes it through a belt loop. "You should do it more. You should get a little bigger."

She tugs that loop when she says "bigger," and my dungarees nearly open for her.

"Let's get a drink," I say, keeping things cool.

"I've got some cold beers in the fridge," she says, looking me straight in the eye.

I think, to hell with catches, and walk beside her for six blocks. She moves like she's got what she wants, like she's pleased with her catch. She smiles and checks me out a few more times before we got to her place. It's small. Fire escapes run up to her third-floor window. She opens it to let in some sun and fresh fall air, and I park myself on the sill.

I hear a tab pulled from the kitchen and she comes out drinking a can of Bud. She tosses me another, and I catch it against my side. It's cold and it wets me.

Putting a boot onto the ledge, I look up at her as she comes close. Saying nothing, she swallows some more beer and pushes my jacket off to the side. She presses a finger into the damp spot on my T-shirt and laughs.

"Gotcha there!" she says. Then she gets playful and

tries to pull my T-shirt up and tag me again with the frosted can. Laughing, I counter with my own and catch her good with a pop-spray to her belly. One glance of the foam trickling from her navel into her jeans is enough to make me want her real bad.

She kisses me, and I taste beer in her mouth. We sit there, making out like school kids for a long time. So smooth. Before I know it, my swollen dick is in her hand, and she's sliding it up and down in her palm. Her nails tickle and scratch at it, making it bigger. I scoop her up and carry her to her bedroom.

"Take off that little thing. I wanna see what you got under there," I tell her.

Her little thermal shirt vanished, and I fixed my gaze on a pair of the roundest, prettiest pair of tits I'd ever seen. I moved close enough to reach out and slide my hands around them, and I watched her smile as I enjoyed their fullness, their utter ripeness.

"Is this what you get from working out?" I laughed.

She squeezed my pecs. "I think I'd prefer something a little beefier in my men!"

There, on our knees, I tugged her jeans down, propped her legs apart, and slid my swollen cock up her muff. Holding each other, pushing into one another, we fucked on the bed like teens in heat. An hour ago, she was checking me out in Washington Square Park—now my dick was being basted in her pussyjuices, and her teeth were sinking into the meat of my shoulder. Pure heaven!

I fucked her until we toppled over, and then we

fucked some more. I don't think we even knew each other's names, but nonetheless we were fucking in her bedroom. Man, was she enjoying it!

When I realized I was getting close to spilling it, I tried one of my old tricks: I pushed myself into her pussy as hard as I could. Nice and slow, mind you, but really hard, so the bottom of my belly is smacking those pussylips of hers. Then I give her a nice, hard grind. The kind that shoves my cock just an inch or two deeper, forcing her clit to shudder against the pressure.

"Ohhhhyyyyeaahhhh!"

Bingo! I got her. I do this a few more times, deep-fucking her brains out, backing up my cock with about a hundred eighty pounds of man-force.

There was so much pressure built up, her come almost squirted out of her pussy! She was screaming so loudly and clawing me so badly, I thought I'd been picked up by a werecat! Finally, I pulled out and shot my load across her belly, laying down seven stripes of gleaming semen, long enough to run right over the hills of her perfect tits and nick the bottom of her pretty chin.

"So what gym do you belong to?" I smiled at her.

"The Washington Square Y," she answered. "As in, why don't you shut up and do that again!"

CAGED HEAT
Will Schwartz

Alexis jumped off her white stallion and went to get a drink of water. She had done enough training for the day and looked forward to the evening off. The tights she wore outlined every inch of her well-muscled legs. The snug, elastic fabric hugged each taut cheek of her ass and outlined the crack of her pussylips. She wasn't very tall, but she was well-proportioned, with hazel eyes and a mane of black hair. Sipping her water, she sauntered over to the lion tamer.

"Damien," she said in her soft, Argentine-accented voice, "how are your pussycats?"

"They're hungry Alexis. Would you like to feed them?" He pointed at a piece of raw steak.

"I'm not as courageous as you, Damien. I'll stick to my horses."

Damien threw a few pieces of steak in the cage and watched the big cats run to their food.

"I could use a bite to eat myself," Alexis murmured.

"Let's go back to my trailer. I'll make dinner for us both!" Damien replied.

Throwing an arm around her shoulders and making small talk, Damien led Alexis to his trailer. It smelled of musk and men's cologne. Knowing full well what was going on, and game for the chase, Alexis went to him immediately and sank to her knees. She took the waistband of his tights and began to slide them off. They fit like a second skin. She rolled the stretchy fabric down over his ass and paused to brush the palm of her hand across his hard behind. It felt every bit as good as she'd ever thought.

Sliding the leggings down toward his ankles, she ran her fingers over his well-shaped thighs, and felt the muscles contract beneath her fingertips. He stepped out of the tights and stood there staring down at her with an awe-inspiring erection-in-progress.

She took all of it into her mouth, licking up the shaft and around the uncut head. He stood motionless, drawing his breath as deeply as if he were performing at the height of his career, and his ass clenched itself into something on the order of marble. She kissed his inner thighs and moved back up slowly, burying her face into his hanging balls.

Damien cupped her face in his powerful hands and pulled her head back. He kneeled in front of her and pulled her spandex top from her lean, supple torso. Her small, firm breasts plopped out, bouncing quickly into place. He leaned down and took her nipples into his mouth and he bit and chewed them. At times he got rough with them, but he seemed to know instinctively when the pain got too severe for her. When that happened, he licked them gently, soothing her with his tongue.

She slipped out of her shiny tights. As he'd always suspected, she wasn't wearing any panties. Touching a finger to the head of his cock, she watched it spring around, tapping against the upper rim of his navel. She was ready for him, and he knew it.

Lying back, she opened herself to him, wrapping her legs around his body. Her pussy was dripping and pulsating, awaiting his phallus eagerly. Holding his cock, he pushed the head inside her and pulled out again. He inserted it again, teasing her a few more times before slowly moving forward. His strokes were long and languid, like the first whispers of air into a toy balloon. As his trade would have indicated, he was a master of control; completely dominant over his own body. Alexis's lips surrounded Damien's, her tongue circling around his, tasting him and reveling in his presence.

Damien held her tightly, thrusting harder and faster. When he came, she could feel the spurting streams of milky sperm inside her twitching body. Indeed, the very sensation of hot come shooting into her throbbing cunt forced her body to begin to spasm. She climaxed with him, a crescendo in this, their latest act, just outside the big top.

They lay in bed together listening to the lions roar in the distance, and the stallions galloping around the ring. She loved the sounds of the circus, and she loved the expertise of the trainers as well.

HOME REPAIRS
Zach Steen

The repairman was supposed to come between 8:00 and 1:00. Well, it was now 2:30 and there was no sign of him. She called the maintenance office, and they told her to be patient. All their men were running late, but someone would be there soon.

At 3:00, the doorbell rang. Boy, was she prepared to give the guy a piece of her mind! But when she saw him, her anger died down. He was tall and very attractive, with broad shoulders, muscular arms, and large hands. She was impressed with his looks. He stepped around her, careful not to hit her with the tool chest he was carrying.

"Where's the damage?" he asked, checking her out.

"Some kids threw a rock through the bedroom window." She didn't take her eyes off him.

She ushered him into the bedroom and watched him while he removed the broken glass skillfully and replaced it with a new pane. He was used to being stared at. He'd long since resigned himself to being an afternoon's entertainment for hundreds of middle-aged women. At least this one was quite a prize, he thought.

Now done with his job, he stood in front of her.

"Is something wrong, ma'am?" He looked her up and down.

"No, you did a great job." She smiled at him.

"Are you as good with your hands on women as you are with your repairs?" she asked demurely.

"I'm very talented with or without my tools." He grinned. "Would you like to find out?"

Without hesitation, she removed her clothes and jumped onto the bed. Following her lead, he unzipped his overalls and tossed them across the room. He had an instant hard-on. She caught it between her lips and pulled a little at the head. Letting go, she blew gently on the tip, then licked at the oozing cockhole. Licking her way down the shaft, she combined her tongue with gentle strokes.

His hands explored her body. They were everywhere—fondling her breasts, tweaking her hardened nipples, stroking her thighs and the crack of her ass. Her flesh felt silky under his rough hands.

He turned her to her side and nibbled her neck and licked her ear. She arched her back and turned her head to kiss him. Lifting her leg up for easy access, he fingered her cunt, checking to see if she was wet enough. He was so hot for her now. Precome had begun to flow out of his cock.

Smearing his thick, massive meat with his own juices, he forced just the head of his cock into her soaking, hot hole.

She moaned and shifted her body to give him freer access. He plunged right in, fucking her wildly, whispering nasty nothings into her ear. He was riding her hard and fast, and she took in his every thrust, lusting for more.

He pulled his dick out and rubbed it between the sweet cheeks of her ass. She got on all fours and teased him by bobbing her butt into his face. He grabbed her hips and, helpless to stop himself, sank his teeth into her plump round cheeks. She yelped, smacking his face, then laughed at his grimace of a reaction.

His cock twitched, still wanting more. He plunged in to the hilt. A loud yell escaped her, and her body stiffened for a second, getting used to the shock of the rear entry. After a few strokes, her hole had loosened a bit. She met every thrust with wild abandon.

He was ramming his cock up her tight hole, fucking her like a dog in heat. He shot his load into her hole while continuing to pump her. His come was oozing out, dripping down her thighs. She reached behind and spread his steamy liquid around her cheeks.

With her sticky fingers, she rubbed her clit and shoved her fingers inside her cunt. As she felt the heat deep inside, she cried out and climaxed, pushing her body into his. He turned her over and licked her pussy clean. She came over and over as he flicked his tongue over her sensitive clit.

They lay in bed, completely wiped out. Suddenly she sprang up and pointed to the bathroom.

"There's a leak under the sink. Can you stop by tomorrow and fix it?" she asked with her hopes up.

"No problem, ma'am. Just call the office and set up the appointment. I'll be here early and stay late just to make sure the job is done right!"

DOCTOR, DOCTOR
Tina Dubois

Nurse Matthews had finished making the hospital bed and was about to walk out of the empty room when Dr. Robbins walked in. Jim Robbins was the talk of the ward. He had the looks of a TV star, and he was often compared to those fiery doctors who seemed to enjoy more time in broom closets than in surgeries. In the case of Dr. Robbins, those hotshot Hollywood television producers had their characters dead-on!

He handed her a chart with her name across the top. This was his little joke. Every time a room was cleared out, he found a reason to detain his favorite nurse. She knew the drill, and heck, why fight it? He was a walking stud.

This time, she was going to be the patient, and he

was going to examine her. He removed her green hospital gown and asked her to take off the rest of her clothes while he watched. In doing so, she tried not to be too "slutty." After all, she was a patient. She folded her nurse's whites on a chair and sat on the bed she'd just made, dutifully waiting for further instructions.

The doctor placed his cold stethoscope on her warm breasts and asked her to breathe deeply. She inhaled and exhaled, sitting straight up as the doctor monitored her heart rate. He then asked her to open her mouth and he held her tongue down with an old-fashioned tongue depressor. His favorite kind.

"Your glands are swollen Ms. Matthews. You need to have your tonsils massaged."

He climbed up on the bed, unzipped his pants, and pulled out his eight-inch cock. He held it in front of her face, tracing her lips with the head, glossing them with traces of precome. She licked the dabs of semen from her lips, and flicked his peehole with the tip of her tongue. Dr. Robbins smiled with approval.

She started gobbling him down, swallowing it whole, determined to be a good patient. Nurse Matthews was very skillful at having her tonsils examined as well as having her tongue depressed at the same time! Her lips found their way to the base of his cock, her teeth just barely scraping the tender flesh. He held her head in position and stroked her hair. She took in just the head and sucked on it before he pushed the shaft all the way in, hitting the back of her throat. Her tonsils already felt much better.

She grabbed his buttocks and pressed her nails into his cheeks. Her hands circled around his ass as she sucked him off, and working her way toward his crack, she found his asshole. Then her finger began to work its way in.

The doctor growled at this new sensation. She buffed his hole nonstop skillfully until the doctor's balls tensed. He had to stop pumping her mouth because he didn't want to come just yet.

He pulled her head away from his cock and flipped her onto her belly. Propping a pillow under her to elevate her ass, he licked his hand and lubed his thick meat with his own spit. Nurse Matthews's pussy was dripping wet.

He prodded her cunt with the enlarged head of his cock, and finally plunged inside. She moaned loudly and pushed her ass toward him to meet his thrusts.

The doctor knew very well how she liked to be fucked. He shoved his pole in and out, punctuating each reentry with a grunt and a hard smack on her ass. The friction of her tight pussy made his cock feel as if it was expanding even more. She felt it twitch like a snake deep inside her snatch.

He grabbed her ass and shoved hard and fast, spilling his warm come. Nurse Matthews howled as she felt his liquid spread upward and then back down as he withdrew, still semihard. Her pussy was throbbing from her climax, but the doctor was not done. He reached between her legs and rubbed her clitoris with the expertise of a man who very damned well knew his anatomy, sending her to new heights of ecstasy.

"I think you'll recover, Ms. Matthews. You're a healthy woman."

"Thank you, Doctor. However I would still like to remain under your care. I'm a firm believer in preventive medicine!"

OPERA APPRECIATION

Jamie Christiansen

Louis slouched down in the box seat next to Tina, his hand on her thigh, almost touching the lips of her pussy. He stroked her there, idly. The only light in the house coming from the stage. The soprano's voice could have broken glass. It ululated across the audience in waves.

He moved his hand up a bit, sliding it over her pussy, finally arriving after a dozen stanzas. Through the light cotton of her panties, he could feel her warmth. He knew she was enjoying this, and he was glad. The tickets to this event had cost him a fortune!

Slowly, deliberately, he began to trace small circles through the fabric over her clit with the tip of his middle finger. She licked her lips and tried hard to keep quiet. Clearing her throat, she shifted in her seat, but

Louis followed every movement she made, and kept up at turning her on.

Tina decided to return the favor. She brushed her fingers across his nuts, sending shivers down his legs and up into his stomach. She brushed them across his crotch and reached under it with her other hand, bunching the looseness of his trousers around his cock and balls.

With her fingers squeezing beneath and her palm applying pressure above, he started getting harder, his engorging cock pressing against the new tightness in his pants. Tina slowly unzipped them and quietly released his engorged meat.

His cock sprang out of his pants as if it had a mind of its own. He shifted again as Tina bent her head over his cock, and he smothered a gasp as her mouth descended over the shaft. First she simply toyed with him, catching his head between her lips, wetting him down with her tongue. But then she engulfed him, eating him up, swallowing him whole.

Abandoning the shaft for a moment, she tilted her head and began to lick and suck at his balls. Shutting his eyes tight, he let the sounds of the opera flow about him and concentrated on the ever-growing hard-on rising higher and higher over his open pants.

He was wondering whether anyone could see Tina's head bobbing up and down—not that he'd really care if they did. The worst they could do was throw them out of this godforsaken opera house!

Her hand was playing with his balls again, rolling them around in her palm. This was just too much for him. He came with a clenching of ass muscles which nearly lifted him out of his seat. It started deep within his balls, and rolled like a wave through his body. Come shot at her, some if it catching in a loose lock of her flaxen hair. Fast losing the struggle to contain himself, he suddenly let fly with a second incredible volley—this one against Tina's sensual lips, coating them both with the warm, sticky mess.

Satisfied with her antics, Tina pulled a silk handkerchief out of her purse and wiped the come off her chin. She then circled it around his shaft and stroked up and down gently, cleaning him up at least enough to prevent unsightly stains at intermission.

Louis smiled at her thoughtfulness and tucked himself back in his pants. They focused on the soprano and sat back in their chairs. Soon Tina felt the comforting weight of his hand once more on her thigh.

LIVING DOLL

Joe Canter

His breathing was quickly getting deeper and faster, and his heartbeat was accelerating. His forehead was glistening with sweat, and he was moistening his lips with his tongue. His steel blue eyes were focused on the petite redhead who was bound tightly to the old wooden chair.

She was completely naked. Her flushed skin was reddened in the areas where the rope dug into her. Her long, silky hair was styled in a ponytail and tied skillfully to the middle slat of the chair's back, pulling her head backward, forcing her to look at the ceiling. Her dark brown eyes were straining, searching to find him. She was very uncomfortable and he knew it.

He walked behind her, bent to her ear and gently nibbled on the meat of her lobe. She could see his shiny, thick silvering hair. He had a musky odor about him, but it was not unpleasant. He dangled a red rubber ball, with leather straps over her face, and watched as her eyes followed the unusual toy as it swayed from side to side. Using an index finger, he forced his way into her mouth.

"Suck on it!" His whisper was a command.

He felt his finger being pulled deep inside her mouth, and her warm tongue circling his rough pointer. He pulled it out and ran it over her luscious lips, making them wet with her own saliva. Then, suddenly forcing her mouth wide open, he stuffed the red rubber ball between her teeth. No longer able to close her mouth or speak, she let out a tiny whimper.

"You're my toy. I own you. I will do whatever I want to you."

He moved behind her, reaching down past her shoulders and grabbing her tits. He squeezed them hard, almost mercilessly. Her helplessness made him smile. She had no choice; she had to look back up at him.

"I've decided not to blindfold you because I want you to see how much pleasure I get by using you." He reached for her large red nipples and gripped them between his thumbs and forefingers. He kept on increasing the pressure until she began to squirm. She was trembling, panting against the pain. Without easing the tension, he began to rub them until they throbbed. They grew swollen and hard, like two jasper pebbles. He was proud of the outcome.

He walked around her and positioned himself in front. He reached inside his button-fly jeans and pulled out his big cock. It was hard, almost beet red. The head was peeking out of the foreskin, and it dripped with precome. He placed his right knee on the chair between her legs, pushing into her wet pussy. Her spread legs strained against their bonds, but they were held fast against the wooden legs of the chair. He leaned down and started chewing on her neck, biting it occasionally. With his right hand, he tugged alternately on her nipples while stroking himself with his left.

"This is only the beginning, my little cunt. This is just a taste of things to come." He pulled and stroked his cock faster and more forcefully. His head fell back. With a deep groan, his cock shot strings of thick white come all over her sore breasts. She felt the hot liquid tingle on her velvety skin and trembled at its warmth.

He breathed deeply, looked down at her and patted her cheek. "You rest for now. I'll come back later...for a little more."

He buttoned his jeans, tucked his shirt in, and walked out of the room, turning the light off before he closed the door.

THE PHOTO SHOOT

Tracy Gustav

She looked stunning, lying in repose on the red velvet couch. Her skin looked positively luminescent, her face framed delicately by her long, silky black hair. His lips yearned to taste her.

He adjusted the lighting in the room and rechecked his light meter, methodically preparing to capture her in just the right way. Focusing the lens of the camera, he snapped exposures at a rate of dozens per moment. Every so often, he asked her to change her pose.

They worked for a couple of hours, then decided to take a break. She lit a cigarette and leaned back on the couch, puffing away as if she hadn't a care in the world. He sat next to her placing an ashtray conveniently on his lap. She looked at it and flashed him a smile.

She leaned forward and tapped a kiss against his temple. He returned the favor by feathering her with a series of light kisses over her cheekbones, down to the tip of her nose, to her chin. Warmth enveloped her whole body. She covered his soft, full lips with hers. Their tongues met and swirled around, exploring the recesses of each others' mouths.

Breaking the kiss finally, he moved to her breasts and began to suckle upon their fat, pointy nipples. Taking first one, then the other, rolling them gently between his teeth, tasting them with his tongue. He licked and nibbled his way down to her pussy and tasted her sweet juices. He flicked his tongue on her clit, making her squirm from the tingling sensations.

His cock was engorged. He rubbed it on the velvet fabric of the sofa preparing it for her cunt. Sensing his need and feeling the same desires, she spread her legs to accommodate him. He positioned himself over her and pressed the head of his cock into her burning, wet pussy. Her bulbous lips surrounded his shaft as he probed deeper inside the depths of her cunt.

He prodded her, using the force of his whole body, enjoying the friction caused by her tightness. He imagined being photographed this way with his model. Her hands were over her head, the top portion of her body completely limp, while she gyrated her hips to a rhythm that matched his.

He stroked in and out, feigning withdrawal occasionally, just to feel the way she would tighten her pussy muscles to keep him from leaving. She put her hands around his neck and lowered his head to meet her lips. She kissed him passionately, holding him firmly as he continued to pound himself into her.

She lifted her hips and ground herself against him, pivoting her body from side to side, forcing him to fill her vagina to overflowing. Her clit was throbbing and her body began to spasm. Her moans filled the room. Her body jerked wildly under his weight. He held her firmly and thrust even faster, making her spring upward with each beefy impact.

Suddenly he stiffened, crying out. His cock leaped, and she felt the warmth of his come shoot waves of liquid heat through her insides. He came for long, intense moments, shooting his balljuice into her again and again.

He stayed hard for a moment or two after his climax, and kept his cock inside her, thrusting a few more times before pulling out. She took his dick gingerly and squeezed it tightly, making him shiver. She blew on it and gave it a quick lick before looking up at him and smiling. He kissed her and then collapsed on top of her sweaty body.

Moments later, he sprang off the couch, picked up his camera, and continued the photo shoot. She lit another cigarette and posed for him as he tried to capture the postorgasmic glow of her flesh on film.

STOCK BOY
Josie Penternast

Joey was in the supermarket basement, checking the inventory for reorders, when his supervisor came up and tapped him on the shoulder. Startled, Joey turned around and shouted, thinking it was his buddy.

"Is that the way to talk to your boss?"

"Sorry, Janet. I thought you were Tony, playing a joke on me."

"I didn't mean to startle you. I came to ask you to open the new cereal shipment and count the product."

He got up to do as he was told. Janet was actually the only person in the store whom he didn't mind asking "How high?" when she said, "Jump." She always wore those tight skirts, silk stockings, and high-heeled shoes. When her smock fluttered open, he'd always steal a glimpse at her large breasts. They were the kind that jiggled with every move. All the stock boys and clerks lusted after her, and she knew it. She actually seemed to enjoy this little routine she had down, ordering them around and standing close to them as they tried to concentrate on their work.

Some of the guys got erections and tried to cover them up from her, but she always seemed to catch them. She'd just smile and walk away, leaving them alone and horny, and usually pretty embarrassed.

Today it looked as if Joey was too cute to be ignored. He had a tanned muscular body, the kind she really got off on. His long legs, tight ass, and thick dark hair weren't half-bad, either, but it was his lips that really sent her over the edge. They were full, with that slight evil curl at the ends. They were the kind of lips that would feel superb lapping at her fresh, warm pussy. She hungered for him, and loved it that the big dummy was completely unaware.

Joey ripped open the first Kellogg's carton and started to count the endless rows of cornflakes boxes inside. Janet walked up behind him and pressed her body against his.

"I think you missed a section," she whispered.

"Hunh?!" He turned around and looked at her, not knowing what to do. "Janet! Wha—?"

She traced his succulent lips with the tip of her tongue, "Why don't you take a little break, Joey-boy. I've been driving you way too hard lately."

Those sweet lips broke into a broad grin, and Joey put his arms around her, pulling her waist to meet his torso. His hand slid down her ass and pushed her lower half against his crotch. His cock was constricted under his tight jeans, but it swelled to proportions bigger than Janet could ever have suspected.

With his teeth, he undid the buttons of her blouse and nibbled on her hard nipples over the fabric of her satin bra. She pulled her skirt over her hips and lowered her pantyhose. As most of the guys in the aisles had speculated correctly, she wasn't wearing any panties.

He slipped his finger between her pussylips and stroked her moist clit. She moaned softly into his mouth, slipping her tongue around his, drawing it into her own. Half-sitting on the stool behind him, Joey unzipped his fly. His stiff cock sprang out and bobbed merrily against her pussy. He placed an arm under her thigh and lifted her leg up and out, giving him access to that all-elusive pussy.

Janet lowered herself onto his erection, her pussy joyously swallowing his thick cockhead before continuing down his shaft. In seconds, she was sitting on him, his dick filling her and growing even bigger within her, probing her deeply.

Joey sat still, letting Janet move her hips up and down on his engorged cock. She found his nipples and suckled them, surprising him, as if no one had ever done that before, making his deep, steady breathing rush.

Suddenly Joey pushed her off his cock and took control. He positioned Janet on all fours down on the floor. He mounted her from behind. With a sudden thrust, he plunged into her cunt, almost knocking her over. She growled and rolled her hips in an attempt to accommodate his hard, fast shoving. The musky scent of her rose to fill the stockroom, and it made him crazy.

"You sure know how to fuck well!" Janet said, between heavy breathing. "Keep on fucking me like this, and I'll promote you to aisle manager, Joey-boy."

He pounded her without saying a word. He didn't care about what she had to say. She could have made him manager of the store! He just wanted to fuck until he came.

Joey took hold of her glossy hair and pulled, causing her back to arch. A sigh escaped her lips, and her rhythm got faster. With his free hand, he fingered her asshole, twisting and turning, making her shudder.

Her body began to shake, and she moaned loudly, her thighs trembling and shivering under the strain. She gasped twice, letting out a high-pitched sigh, before her body finally went limp. He slapped her ass and pumped her cunt, feeling the heaviness build up deep inside his balls.

His ass muscles clenched, his nuts tightened, and he let out a sharp *"Yeah!"* as he shot his wad into her well-fucked hole. He grunted each time he stabbed her cunt, firing all the hot cream he'd built up since he'd jerked off in the shower that morning. It was more than enough!

Janet was pleased with his performance. She planned to make him her personal stock boy and keep him working in the basement alone for as long as she could. As manager, she'd have no trouble, and Joey would be rewarded well whenever he did a good job!

FINE ARTS
Gloria Santiago

The show was opening tomorrow, and Gene was working on last-minute preparations. Trudy was following him around taking notes on things she had to follow up. The artwork had being arranged by theme on the white walls of the gallery. By all accounts, it looked as if they had done a good job.

Gene decided to take a short break. He had a long evening ahead. He sat on the floor in the center of the gallery and studied the artwork. Trudy joined him, and they spent some time gossiping about the patrons who would be coming in tonight. Trudy told him about how Mr. Winston had once confided to her his predilection for being pleasured by female midgets. Gene laughed and fired one back about Ms. Tripplehorn, who refused to make love without her boa constrictor sharing the bed with her men! The conversation soon evolved to the point where the two were discussing their own sexual interests.

Trudy told Gene that she always wondered what it would be like to get fucked on the cold, hard wooden floor of the empty gallery.

"Would you like to find out?" he asked with a smile.

She thought about it for a few seconds and decided to go for it. He was cute enough. Better yet, he was funny! She got up in front of Gene and stripped her clothes off while giddily singing a sexy French song to him. Her voice filled the large room, and she wiggled her ass in his face with every stanza. She whirled her naked body about with so much abandon, her breasts bouncing happily along, that Gene could only gaze with disbelief.

Gene took off his shirt and pants and lay back on the floor, hands behind his head, a big grin on his face, watching her as his penis rose high into the air. She squatted over his head and lowered herself, stopping only inches from his lips. When he reached up to lick her protruding clitoris, Trudy almost leaped away at the electric touch. Instead, she stayed there, moaning and continuing with her song. She sat on his face and let Gene probe her pussy with his tongue.

After she had been lubed thoroughly, she turned around and propped herself in the sixty-nine position. Gene was fully erect now, and Trudy worshiped his prick with her fingers and tongue, licking it as if it were a lollipop, with long wet strokes up and down the shaft.

Then she pulled his cock to one side and placed her lips on his balls, sucking at them gently, rolling them around in her mouth. She licked at the line that divided the sacs, tickling him, turning him on even more. Gene growled and sucked hard on her throbbing clit, making her rub her cunt hard on his face.

She took Gene's thick rod greedily into her mouth once again, almost choking on it. Relaxing her mouth, she opened the back of her throat wide enough to take it all the way down. He slid his cock in and out of her mouth, even as she provided counterpleasure with her own lips and tongue. She could feel his precome oozing out of his cock slit and dribbling down her gullet. The taste was not at all unpleasant!

Gene flipped Trudy over on her back, raised her knees, and pushed her thighs apart. He buried his face in the crack of her ass and licked at the hole. She moaned loudly and stroked his hair in return. He took the precome from the tip of his cock onto his fingers and lubricated her opening. With his prick in his hand he guided the head toward her tight hole, and pushed it in slowly. Trudy shook her head from side to side in a mixture of agony and ecstasy.

He moved within her, tight circles pulling out of the tight opening again and again, thrusting harder and harder with every reentry. Trudy massaged her clit vigorously, shouting with ecstasy as she took Gene's lunges.

She tensed and gave in to the waves of intense pleasure that rippled throughout her body. He felt her contractions as her asshole tightened around his rock-hard dick. Increasing his rhythm, feeling the tension deep within his balls, he grunted a loud counterpoint to her shouts. And with each of his last several thrusts, he exploded jets of milky white jism, filling her up to the point of bursting!

The release had been intense. He pulled out and collapsed on the floor next to her, his body absorbing the coolness of the polished wooden boards.

Though the break had certainly been longer than intended, they didn't really care. They'd worked hard enough!

"I wonder whether I should confide this to Mr. Winston," Trudy said with a touch of irony.

"Why not? Just tell him you did it with a male midget. It might inspire him to buy a few paintings!"

They chuckled and lay in each other's arms.

EMERGENCY BRAKE
Mitch Slovak

It was after midnight on the downtown express train, and I was riding with my girlfriend Daphne. We were slumped in each other's arms in the corner two-seater, engaged in idle chitchat. The car was empty except for one other guy reading the paper at the far end.

The fluorescent lights were flickering overhead, the train was traveling at top speed, and I decided to kiss Daphne. Her lips tasted of sweet cherries from the Slurpie she had just finished. I licked some of the sweetness off. She tried to get it back, and our tongues wrestled. We giggled and poked each other. Suddenly the train came to a screeching halt. We almost fell out of our seats. The guy at the other end was startled.

We were stuck in a subway tunnel. A voice came over

the static-filled loudspeaker, and announced that the emergency brake had been pulled by vandals, and we'd be moving in about twenty minutes. Since there was nothing we could do, we resumed our kissing. What better way was there to spend the time?

Daphne's hand traveled down my torso, down my abs, and stopped at my engorged bulge. I could feel her lips breaking into a smile, happy with her discovery. She pressed on it gently and rubbed my aching cock.

With a feathery touch, I ran my fingers down the side of her neck, stopping at the center of her cleavage. I unbuttoned her shirt and slipped one hand down her warm chest. Her tits were full and round, her tender flesh spilling slightly over the cups of her tight satin bra. I rubbed the tips of my fingers across her hard, protruding nipples. A low moan escaped her lips. Her body shuddered at my touch.

My cock was pressing firmly against my denims. Daphne unhooked my waistband button and stuck her hand down my pants. She located my swollen, throbbing cockhead and caressed it with her fingers. I couldn't stand the pressure any longer. I unzipped my jeans and let my cock bounce out.

"What are you doing? He'll see us!"

"So? What is he gonna do—report us to the police? Just relax and play with it, babe."

She didn't need any more convincing. My cock twitched and bobbed back and forth as she stroked the underside of the shaft. She massaged my sac delicately, rolling my balls between her palms. Her hands gripped it at the base. Increasing the pressure and the tempo, she jerked and tugged, pushing out precome from pulsing muscle.

"Get up and stand in front of me!"

I followed her instructions reluctantly. Her lips surrounded the head and, very slowly, she sucked the rest of my long, thick member all the way into her mouth. One of her hands kneaded my balls while the other gripped my shaft. Her tongue twirled around and her head pumped back and forth without skipping a beat.

I was supporting myself on the chrome bar overhead, one foot resting on the seat next to her, thrusting my hips forward. It seemed as though she was in a trance—sucking my dick was her only focus. She pushed my cock up the top of her mouth with her tongue and increased the suction, creating more friction. I couldn't stand it any longer. My blood was boiling. My balls tensed, and pushed the weight of my hot come with such explosive force that streams of milky liquid shot into Daphne's welcoming mouth.

Suddenly, the train began to move. Almost losing my balance, I dropped down into the seat. My whole body was limp. I was breathing deeply, and I could feel my heart pounding in my chest.

Daphne was wiping off her mouth, and I was relaxing, with my dick hanging out. The train finally pulled into our stop. I tucked myself in, took Daphne's hand, and we waited for the doors to open.

"So long, folks. Thanks for the show! I'll tell ya—it

was a whole helluva lot better than reading the *Wall Street Journal!*"

Daphne and I had forgotten all about the other passenger. As the doors opened, we waved to him and ran out giggling. We had a great time being stuck in the tunnel. Apparently, so did our friendly spectator!

THE BARMAID
Jerry Cohen

It was noon, and Jackie had just opened the bar a few moments earlier. No one had come in yet except for Andy, the cleaning boy; and he was out back, prepping the beer drums for the tap. She was wiping down the counter when Hank walked in. Hank was the owner of the sport shop across the street, and stopped by every day for a scotch and soda and a chat with Jackie. They liked each other, but never went further than a drink and light conversation at the bar.

"Place needs cheering up," he said, throwing a quarter into the jukebox and punching up a country-western melody.

He sat down. Without asking, Jackie placed his drink in front of him with a bowl of peanuts. Hank took a sip and winked at her. Jackie blew him a kiss and returned to setting up.

"How's it going, doll-face?"

"Okay, I guess. It's been slow the last couple of weeks. I'm thinking of taking some time off, maybe rent a house near the beach for about a week."

Hank took a sip and checked out her body. She was tall and slim, with shoulder-length straight hair. Still young. Good curves to her. She always wore tight outfits—she made more tips that way, he reckoned—and high heels, no matter how many hours she had to stand. Her nails were polished red, and she wore rings on almost every finger. Hank was very attracted to Jackie. If he had to admit it, she was the only reason he came in every day.

"Hey, Jackie, I want to talk with you in private. You think that Andy could watch the bar for a few minutes?"

Jackie gave Hank a perplexed look. She knew that if he made that request of her, it must be serious. She wiped her hands, called Andy to the front, and told him she'd be back in a few minutes. She took Hank into the bar's office, and they sat on the worn-out couch.

"What's up, Hank?"

"I just want to let you know that I really like you, and I was wondering if you would be interested in going to dinner or maybe a movie with me."

They sat there for a while in silence. Hank felt nervous, preparing to apologize and call it off, when Jackie leaned over and kissed him deeply, pushing her tongue between Hank's teeth, thrusting herself into his mouth. It took about ten seconds for Hank to get over the shock. Then he responded to Jackie's kiss.

After long minutes of heavy kissing, Jackie placed her hand on Hank's crotch. His cock beneath the bleached denims, reared up to fill Jackie's hand. As Jackie opened Hank's fly, his heavy penis grew right out of it, falling neatly into Jackie's waiting hands. She bent her head over Hank's cock and covered him with her mouth. Hank's head fell back as his trousers struck the floor, and he felt Jackie's tongue circle the shaft, delivering wet caresses beyond anything he'd ever felt before.

Jackie ran the rough part of her tongue down the underside of Hank's rod, and across the balls nestled underneath. She took one between her lips and ran the tip of her tongue in tight circles across the twin sacs. Going lower, she spread the cheeks of Hank's ass and licked around the tight hole, probing it with the tip of her tongue.

Hank's breath came in short, agonized gasps. Jackie looked up at Hank and grinned, going again for his cock, taking him whole. Suddenly Jackie shoved a long index finger up Hank's ass, stretching the tightness a bit, working her finger around the opening and probing deeper, massaging Hank from the inside.

"Good Lord! Jesus Christ, you're a wild one, Jackie!"

Hank groaned as Jackie started sucking his cock again, applying pressure with her lips while using the tip of her tongue just at the head. Finally, with one last thrust of her fingers up Hank's ass, Jackie raised her head.

Hank's balls contracted. It seemed to Jackie as if Hank's entire cock backed up before shooting streams of hot come onto her full cleavage. Jackie pumped Hank's cock with her hand, milking it of every last drop. Then, as Hank lay there on the sofa, Jackie went into the bathroom, got a washcloth, and cleaned Hank off.

"Does that mean yes?" Hank asked Jackie.

"I would love to go out with you, Hank. I just wanted to do this for a while now. Didn't have the patience to wait till after our date. Hope you don't mind?"

Hank smiled and kissed her. "Not at all, doll. Scotch and soda with a blowjob chaser is more than I could hope for. You're gonna wind up spoiling me."

"I love to spoil my men. Now I gotta get back before Andy starts to wonder." She blew him a kiss and walked out front to her counter.

AUTO REPAIR SHOP
Vinnie Petrocelli

Lily waited impatiently as the mechanic tinkered under the hood of her Ford, trying to determine what the problem was. Every minute he was under that hood meant about ten dollars more draining into the old wreck. By this point, her mood was drifting into seriously pissed off.

After a while, the mechanic popped his head up and smiled at his customer. She was a pleasant sight. "You're gonna need to replace your air filter and your spark plugs."

"How long will that take?" She didn't know whether to be irritated or relieved. He looked cute, though, with that touch of motor grease on his nose.

"Not long. You can wait while I do the job," he answered.

She didn't really want to linger in that greasy cesspool, but the shop was located in an industrial area. There was nowhere else to go. She walked around the shop for a few moments. Everything was covered in grime—even the voluptuous asses on the girls in the tool calendar were smeared with oil. In fact, the only thing worth more than a passing glance in the whole garage was this polite mechanic's coverall-covered butt. She stood by his side, watching his every move.

She realized that she enjoyed watching him handle her engine with his muscular hands. She stared at his broad shoulders and imagined what they'd look like if they were bare. Idle thought drifted into active fantasy, and she felt a stirring in her loins just thinking about his greasy hands feeling her up.

At that moment, he looked up at her and asked her if she'd feel better sitting inside the car. She watched his lips move, not listening to his words.

"This may take longer than I thought," he said.

"Yeah, okay," she murmured.

He smiled, wiped his hands on his coveralls, and stepped closer. "Are you all right?"

"Huh? Oh, yeah, I'm just fine." She regained control of her senses and decided to throw an ace.

She reached out and touched his biceps.

"They're so big and muscular!" The dumb-blonde routine. It worked every time.

He reached out and traced the line of her face with the tips of his fingers. They were rough and callused, and she could smell motor oil on them. He touched her lips, and she parted them. Grinning now, he pulled her close to him and kissed her.

Lily felt his hard-on pressing against her, and she moaned softly into his mouth. His kisses were deep and tender. It surprised her that such a tough-looking guy could be so gentle. She forgot about her surroundings quickly and allowed her physical desires to overtake her.

She located the zipper of the mechanic's coveralls and pulled it down. Slipping her hands inside, she swept her palms over his torso, feeling the hard contours of his muscles. Without letting go of her lips, he unbuttoned her blouse. He undid her bra releasing her full, round breasts. He cupped them both and massaged them gently, flicking her nipples lightly.

Lily's hands traveled downward, purposely scraping his flesh with her nails. She stopped when the tip of his swollen head touched her palm, and she felt his precome ooze from his dickhole. Grasping his shaft, she squeezed it firmly, pushing down and pulling up.

Kneeling down in front of him, Lily freed his cock and took all eight inches of it into her greedy mouth. She encased the head with her lips and sucked on it, circling the rim with her tongue. She licked up and down the shaft, occasionally nipping and gently biting on it. She pulled it out of her mouth and focused on his sensitive sacs.

He slid his hands under her arms and pulled her up. He lifted her skirt over her hips, turned her around, and bent her over the hood of her car. With his rough hands, he kneaded her ass, making her spread her legs instinctively and rise up on her toes, butt high up in the air.

The mechanic licked his finger and stuck it up her drenched cunt, moving it in and out slowly, massaging her from the inside. He pulled his finger out. Then, without warning, he plunged his monster cock inside, pushing it up to the hilt. A wail escaped her lips.

His hands held fast to her hips, setting the rhythm, almost withdrawing entirely before slamming back in again. He knocked the breath out of her with every thrust. Leaning on her elbows, she clenched her fists as she felt the pressure build up. She wiggled her ass even as her pussy contracted, sending shock waves of ecstasy, each one escaping in the form of loud moans.

The mechanic drove into her one final time before he stiffened. His cock erupted within her, spilling his hot, creamy jism into her climaxing pussy. The milky liquid backed up and ran down his dick, soaking both thatches of pubic hair in a pungent glaze.

Still gasping, he wiped the come off her legs with his hands, and rubbed it all around her plump ass. She felt his sweat trickle on her back. He had given her quite a lube job, she mused. He pulled out his dick and turned her around, kissing her one last time, pushing the hair away from her face. She looked satiated.

"Would you mind checking my brakes. Also the steering fluid, and maybe the transmission. The car may even need a wheel alignment. Oh, and don't forget the carburetor!" She whispered in his ear.

SALES REP

Jim Fraenkle

"Hi, Len." Christa motioned him into her office. "You're early."

Len shrugged shyly at the buyer and entered. Christa was one of the friendlier buyers in this department store, but he still felt a little nervous around her. With her endless legs and power suits, those huge green eyes, and that amazing jet-black hair, she was a knockout. To top it off, he thought she liked him!

"What do you have to show me today?" she asked.

"I-I have a new line of perfumes and body lotions," Len almost stammered. "This is our new spring product. The scent is light and fresh, with a hint of wildflowers."

He opened his duffel bag and pulled out the delicate glass bottles, placing each one carefully on her desk.

Christa sampled a few, finding it difficult to decide which one she liked best.

"And now I want to show you the lotions. These are gentle for all skin types and they moisturize, too." He pulled out a tall plastic bottle, opened the cap, and squirted a dab into her palm. Christa rubbed it up and down her arm, enjoying the silky feeling.

"This feels good, Len." She got up from her chair. "Would you mind rubbing some on my back?"

Len couldn't believe his ears! Christa turned her back to him and removed her blouse and her bra. He squirted the lotion in his hand, rubbed his palms together, and smoothed it on the firm flesh of her back. She moaned and shrugged her shoulders.

"Y-You're sure this is okay, C-Christa?"

"Len, don't be such a baby!" she cooed.

There was simply no way Len could stop himself from getting a hard-on. He slipped his hands towards the front and cupped her breasts. Her tits were small, but plump and bouncy. Her nipples were erect. She leaned back on him and ground her ass into his stiff cock. He pressed it between her crack, and continued playing with her nipples.

Christa turned around and kissed Len on the lips. He pushed the mass of perfume bottles to the side and lifted her onto the desk. He removed her shoes and pulled off her dress slacks. Her lace panties were damp at the crotch from her juices. He traced her pussylips over the lace in minute circles, making her shudder at his touch. To her surprise, he tore her panties off and flung them across the room.

"I won't be a baby anymore!" he smiled.

He lifted her legs up and pushed them back, exposing her hungry cunt. With one hand he unhooked his belt quickly, pulled down the zipper, and let his pants drop to the floor. His stiff cock was standing at attention, ready for the plunge. He grabbed the shaft tightly and prodded her clit with the thick cockhead. Her pussy was soaked. He positioned the head at the opening and pushed hard, penetrating the wet, tight hole.

He pushed his body up against hers, feeling her hard nipples poke at his torso. Her scent was mixing perfectly with the wildflower perfume, and it made him giddy with lust. He probed her mouth with his fingers, and she sucked on them as if they were little penises, twirling her tongue around each one, biting down gently on them.

He fucked her hard, slamming his body into hers with every push. She was getting massaged inside and out. Her moans made him even more excited.

She dug her nails into his back and held on, pushing her hips up for maximum impact. He fucked her harder and faster, licking and sucking on her neck. She began to moan louder and louder, jerking her body beneath his. Len felt her body squirm and shudder under his, but he continued to pump without skipping a beat.

He rammed his cock fast and furious, feeling the pressure build up in his scrotum. The sweat was trickling down his face and dripping on her torso. She found his nipples and pinched them with her long red nails. He clenched the muscles of his ass, his balls tightened and, at last, he shot his creamy load into her throbbing cunt. He pulled out quickly and let the remainder of his come drip onto her belly. He smeared it all around, mixing it with the body lotion he had applied only moments earlier.

"I like the smell of wildflowers and jism combined," Christa laughed.

"Maybe I can bottle it up."

"I'll help you produce the come," she smiled and stroked his semihard cock, not wanting to let go.

THE PICNIC
Trish Boscovich

They lay down on the grass, soaking in the sun. Allan unbuttoned Marie's cotton sweater, exposing her bare breasts beneath it, his fingers grazing her skin in the process. Allan's fingers felt warm against her flesh.

Allan kissed her deeply, his tongue flirting with Marie's as he pulled down the zipper of her jeans. Marie wiggled her hips and legs as Allan pulled off her denims. He kissed his way down, pausing at the nipples, licking and sucking at them until they were erect. Marie shuddered.

He trailed her tummy with his tongue, pausing at her navel and exploring its depth. He continued downward until he reached her mound. He grabbed a tuft of pubic hair with his lips and tugged gently. He could smell the musky scent of her pussy, and it aroused him. He pushed her soft thighs apart disclosing her moist pink clit. He poked at it with the tip of his tongue, making her writhe at the touch. Her pussy was saturated with her juices.

Suddenly Marie pushed Allan backward with her legs. She jumped over him and undid the buttons of his jeans. His stone-hard cock sprang out, ready to take her on. She grabbed the bottom of the shaft holding it straight up and took him whole, working her tongue up the shaft from bottom to head. She traced the rim. Then Allan's cock disappeared into her mouth again. Her lips caressed it as her tongue twirled side to side on the shaft. She cupped his sac, gently pulling and massaging it, occasionally slipping her tongue over the tender spheres.

After a few minutes, she pulled Allan's engorged prick out of her mouth and, in a few quick movements, mounted it. She slid down his meaty pole, sheathing it with her damp cunt, and then pounced on his erection as if she were riding a wild bull.

He grabbed her tits and pulled them into his mouth, suckling vigorously on them. She was grunting and growling, completely lost in rapture. Then, just as quickly, Allan flipped her over and pinned her hands on the ground over her head. The surprise of his actions turned her on even more causing her to explode, her body trembling as she came.

The head of his cock found its own way to the entrance of Marie's contracting pussy and, within seconds, was shoving itself home. He withdrew almost completely, and then lunged back in again. He slammed hard and fast into her, knocking the wind out of her.

Finally Allan planted himself deeply, tightened his ass muscles, and fired several powerful shots of hot come, lathering Marie's cunt. He held his position until he was completely spent, and then pulled out to lie on top of her naked body.

Relishing the feel of the wind sweeping across their bare skin, they listened to the birds chirp and watched the overgrown grass sway back and forth. The bright hot sun bathed their bodies, and they quietly dozed off in each other's arms as the ants busily smuggled bits and pieces of their sandwiches underground.

LOONY WARD
Cynthia Freeley

It was lights-out on the late shift at the hospital, and all the patients on the psycho ward had been secured and locked down. The guards had gone on tour, and the nurse at the receptionist's desk sipped coffee and went over the day's records.

Just on her first break, Francine sneaked into the supply closet for a smoke. She stood there taking a deep drag off the cigarette, enjoying the burning sensation of the smoke filling her lungs. It soothed her.

She heard footsteps right outside the door. She stubbed out the cigarette as the door opened. Waving the smoke from the air with her hand, she turned to face the intruder. It was Nick, the orderly.

Nick was a sweet and naturally gorgeous guy. He had a muscular physique from his daily workouts. It was important for an orderly to be strong in this hospital, and Nick was rarely remiss in his duties. He also always seemed to know where she was hanging out, and tracked her down like a bloodhound. She didn't mind because they smoked the same brand of cigarettes and shared a sick sense of humor.

He locked the door behind him and placed a finger to his lips. He came closer and, to her surprise, feathered a light kiss on the tip of her nose. He removed her lab coat, still not saying anything. He put his arms around her and unzipped her dress, letting it fall to the floor. She was alarmed but excited. She knew she could trust him.

After he had folded the dress and put it neatly on a shelf, he opened a package of gauze, took her wrists, and tied them over her head to the steel shelves. Now she was amused, wondering what he would do next. His warm fingers brushed the skin on her stomach as he removed her panties carefully and pulled them down around her ankles. With his foot, he pushed her legs apart gently.

He stood face to face with her and grinned. He was holding two pairs of disposable forceps. He opened one and hooked it onto one of her hard nipples. She gasped at the sudden pain. When he did the same thing to the other one, she bit her lower lip to keep from crying out. Francine felt a wave of dizziness.

"Nick—that's too painful!" she hissed through her teeth.

He just placed his finger against her luscious red lips

and, without saying a word, continued with his plan. He spread her pussylips apart and tickled her clit. The combination of pleasure and pain had her standing on her tiptoes, gasping for breath.

Nick dropped to his knees and began to lick her cunt. His tongue danced around the tip of her clit, teasing her. Without warning, he plunged his finger in and out of her asshole. Between his mouth and finger, Francine started to moan a little too loudly. Her clit was throbbing under the onslaught of Nick's lips and tongue.

It was sweet agony not to be able to touch him. Nick would decide when Francine could actually lay her hands on his body.

He kept tracing every wrinkle and fold of her cunt and asshole with his tongue and the sharp edges of his teeth, until her juices were pouring out of her pussy like water from a faucet.

Suddenly Nick thrust three fingers up her tight pussyhole and pushed and turned, until her body twisted and shook as if she were a rag doll. Francine was biting her lips to keep from screaming; only garbled moans managed to escape. Her climax was strong and intense. Her fluids drenched his hand.

Nick untied her wrists, removed the clamps from her nipples—which gave her a rush of renewed pain—and held her in his arms, feeling the warmth of her naked body. He kissed her lips and told her that it was time for her to thank him.

Francine dropped to her knees and took his stiff cock into her mouth.

She sucked hard simultaneously yanking his shaft and squeezing his balls gently. Tracing every part of him with her tongue, repeating her motions in a quickening rhythm, she was getting him more excited than he'd been before. Before too long, Nick felt a profound heaviness deep within his balls, traveling up the shaft of his cock until it exploded from the tip, coating Francine's hands and wrists in hot, steaming sperm. She shoved his dick into her mouth quickly, sucking him dry.

She grinned up at him and wiped her face on his sleeve. She stood up and kissed his lips, and they embraced that way for several minutes, enjoying each other's scent.

After a few moments, they got dressed. Their break was over, and they were due back on their posts in less than a minute. They looked at their watches, and as they hurried out of the closet Francine reminded Nick that their next break was in four hours. Nick winked at her and told her that there was an empty room on the third floor. She smiled at him and walked away, thinking of all the possibilities.

THE TENANT
Gary Benderfield

His landlady had been patient so far, but she had warned him about being late with the rent money last time. Things were looking pretty grim.

"Mr. Jordan, it's Ms. Stroeber." There was a tapping at his door. "I need to speak with you."

His heart skipped a beat. How could such a sweet voice—and sexy body—belong to such a cold person? What was he going to tell her? Too late now. He opened the door and offered her a weak smile.

"Mr. Jordan, it's the fifteenth of the month. I simply cannot wait for the cash any longer!"

"Jeez, I'm sorry, Ms. Stroeber. Ever since I lost my job, it's been so difficult for me to make ends meet. Is there any other way that I can repay you? Maybe I can do some odd jobs around the building?"

"Well, I don't like to make a habit out of it, but I guess we can arrange something." She adjusted her glasses and licked her glossy lips thoughtfully. "I already have a handyman, but there is something else you can do for me."

"Anything! Just name it and I'll do it!"

"Great!" Her gorgeous face was stony, her mind made up. "I want you to remove your clothes and lie on your bed. Don't ask any questions—just do it."

He was puzzled by her request, but followed her instructions.

"Now stroke your cock until it's good and hard. Look at me while you're doing it."

He grabbed the shaft, pulled hard on it, and let go. His cock was enormous. It hung between his legs, its massive weight supported by his balls. He pulled and let it drop again, but it started to come back up by itself.

Cool and collected, she unbuttoned her blouse slowly. Her breasts were very large, with enormous dark pink nipples. The idea of his landlady seducing him this way was outrageous. She'd always been so indifferent to him, he hadn't even fantasized about something like this. His cock hardened at the sight of her luscious breasts. He couldn't wait to taste them.

"Well, what are you waiting for? Come suck on them!"

He sprang from the bed, grabbed her by the waist, and pulled her into him. For a second he just looked at her, greedily, taking in her perfectly pinned hair, those delicate features, that air of perfumed rigidity. Then he plunged his face into her big milky white tits, and took as much of them as he could into his hungry mouth. For long moments, he sucked on each large pink nipple like a starving baby.

She placed her hand at the back of his head, as if to support him while he was feeding busily. She lowered her free hand to his huge erection and cupped the plum-shaped head, feeling him push himself into her palm. It was more than ready.

"Sit on the edge of the bed, Mr. Jordan."

She watched him carefully as he backed up and sat down. She turned around, facing away from him, and lifted her long flared skirt, exposing a plump, round ass.

"Hold your cock straight up for me, Mr. Jordan."

She lowered herself onto his massive hardness, allowing a barely audible gasp as she felt him enter her soaked cunt. He pulled her asscheeks apart and rubbed her hole vigorously. The only clue he had about how she felt about this was the fact that her breath seemed to come a bit more quickly.

Before long, she was bouncing on his cock with a steady certainty. She was enjoying herself, almost as if he weren't there! He could feel her wet, burning cunt tightening around his shaft as she approached her climax. He was sure she was.

He reached his hand around her front and found her clit. With his index and middle finger, he tweaked it as fast as he could. She tensed her legs, and, barely losing her perfect posture, began trembling violently on his towering pole.

His cock drowned in her cuntjuice, but she stayed steady, allowing him to continue on, pushing his cock in and out of her. He felt the walls of her pussy throbbing. No, he thought. He was going to get a rise out of her yet!

He put his fingers near her nose.

"Smell your pussy, Ms. Stroeber."

"It tastes as good as it smells," he whispered, parting her lips and sliding his fingers into her mouth. "Suck on them and taste your pussyjuices, Ms. Stroeber."

At first she moved almost imperceptibly. But soon she was sucking on his fingers, allowing them to explore her mouth.

"Suck hard, Ms. Stroeber. Pretend you have a cock in your mouth and make it come."

She sucked, nibbled, and even tried to swallow his fingers.

"Aw, man! I can't hold it anymore. I'm gonna come!"

He gave her three last, rough strokes and then he blew up inside her. She felt the warm liquid fill her, and then she felt it ooze out.

He lifted her from him, placed her back down on his bed, spread her legs apart, and drank his come from her dripping cunt. She moaned at the touch of his lips on her sore pussy. After he sucked every last bit, he moved up to face her. He held her head gently and kissed her, giving her a taste of their passion.

"By the way," she interrupted, "this does not include late charges!"

SWIMMING LESSONS
Ben Torres

Louisa walked into the pool room wearing a shiny red high-cut spandex bathing suit. It clung to her body, accentuating every curve. Her magnificent breasts, with their protruding pointy nipples, beckoned to me. She had long lean legs with a full derriere. Her suit was tight enough to have slipped a bit. It bunched at her crack.

It was very difficult trying to concentrate on giving her swimming lessons. She was one of my best students, but I got nervous every time I had to get close to her, to show her the proper techniques. Today she had booked a private lesson with me. She was determined to improve her style by the beginning of the summer, or so she said.

She dove into the water and swam towards me rising up, all wet, to greet me.

"Good morning, Mr. Armstrong," she said with a big smile.

"Good morning, Louisa. Ready for your lesson today?"

"I can't wait to get started, but it feels like my leg is about to cramp up. Think you could help me work out the kink?" she asked with a slight pout.

She hoisted herself up onto the concrete side of the pool and lifted her leg up to me. I began to rub her silky-smooth leg with my thumbs in circles. I could see the line the spandex of her suit was making over her pussy, as she sat with her legs slightly parted. She tilted her head back and moaned softly as I applied pressure.

"Mr. Armstrong, you're so good, I'd love to get a full-body massage from you sometime."

"Anything for my number-one student!"

She gave me a long look and she removed her straps off her shoulders and pulled down the top of her bathing suit. Her tits plopped out, glistening from the water. Her nipples were large and dark.

She cupped her breasts and tugged her nipples gently, making them erect. I could feel my erection growing.

She reached at my torso and rubbed it with her toes...then, suddenly, she slid into the water, placing her arms around my shoulders. She gave me a deep, long kiss. I could feel her hard nipples rubbing against my chest. I reached around her waist and removed her bathing suit. With that, she wrapped her legs around me and thrust her cunt against my groin.

She lowered a hand under water and touched the

head of my cock with her finger. I drew in a breath, letting it out slowly. She folded her hand around my cock and began to draw her fingers up and down the shaft, circling the head with her thumb. Her eyes closed as she felt me expanding in her hand.

I was at full attention when she let go and pressed against me. I felt the softness of her belly. She rubbed up and down, creating friction for my rockhard cock. I pushed her against the tile wall of the pool and spread her legs apart and over my arms. I braced my hands behind her on the edge of the pool and pushed myself in her tight, yearning cunt.

I began a gentle stroking motion, pushing in and out slowly, the weight of the water keeping me from going faster. Each thrust was punctuated by the sounds of lapping water and her soft moans of pleasure. She leaned toward me and gave me her tongue. Her natural taste mixed with the chlorinated water. She slipped her tongue around mine, pushing her hips to meet my every thrust.

She grabbed the back of my hair and pulled, biting my lips, jerking her body forward. She growled into my mouth, her sweet breath rushing in making my head spin. Her orgasm was powerful. She clenched her legs tightly around me as her body continued to spasm.

I couldn't hold back any longer. I felt the pressure deep within my balls, and I was grunting loudly as I pumped her. I came, spurting jism deep within her, filling her up. Some of my creamy liquid seeped out and floated to the top. I reached back, grabbed her by the waist, and pulled her in, holding her there, tightening my own asshole as much as I could, then loosening it again, making sure I was completely drained.

We held each other for a couple of moments, and then we let go. We pushed away from the wall and floated on our backs, allowing the cool water to soothe our tired bodies.

STUDENT UNION
Griffin Edmund

She was a black-maned beauty with big dark eyes and a body that just would not quit. She had somehow managed to tan her skin a light golden, though June had not yet arrived. The white of her blouse and her cheerful smile shone incredibly against it. She turned toward me as the song changed in the rathskeller, and I danced with her.

Tossing her hair, grinning and swinging her hips to the rhythm, she truly seemed to be enjoying herself, and certainly not minding me. I could not help noticing her breasts as they jiggled beneath the sheer silky fabric of her blouse. They were perfectly rounded, creamy, pert, capped with high nipples, which had begun to protrude. She wore a pair of tight white designer jeans which hugged each of her strong thighs—each healthy asscheek—like the skin of a ripe grape.

As she swayed, her shirt shimmered in the blue neon, puckering about her torso, fluttering over the denim of her pants everywhere except where they buttoned tightly over her lower belly. The look of it pulled my eyes and thoughts lower.

A slow song brought us together. She hugged me close, her hands running down the length of my back, feeling the firmness of my musculature through my shirt, from my shoulders to my ass. She squeezed me and my crotch rubbed squarely into hers in time with the music. I was becoming aroused, and she didn't seem to mind.

Her body was lean and strong in my arms. I could tell she'd been taking special care of herself. I invited her up to the club office on the second floor. To my delight, she took my hand and went up with me.

Her tongue was soft and sweet in my mouth. She seemed to enjoy kissing me and did so there in the darkness, until she finally broke away to undo the buttons of my shirt. With the tip of her tongue, she licked the edge of my ears, nuzzled my throat and curled around my pecs.

Rubbing my erection with the palm of her hand through the denim, she pulled the tails of my shirt aside to gently tug my jeans open. The pop of the snap echoed in the silence, and as she began to unzip them she ran her moist, velvety tongue over the six-pack abs of my belly. Folding down the front of my jeans, she then took my completely engorged penis, expertly slid it into her mouth until it seemed to reach deeply down her throat, and pulled on it with a nod, wetly and lovingly.

With her hands around my thighs and her fingertips trailing over the warm crook of my ass, she fellated me until I was on the verge of an exquisite orgasm. Then she stopped and looked up at me, eyes shining, glossy lips smiling beautifully. She wanted me to explode inside that gorgeous, unstoppable, sexy body of hers. I told her that I would be only too happy to do just that.

I leaned her down on the desk, upon which I'd played Rummy-Q and rolled joints with my buddies. I pulled those white jeans off her long legs and tossed them in the shadows, like a faint ghost. I got up over her and pushed myself slowly, evenly into her. A soft, easy moan escaped her, and I pushed my lips into hers as we began to fuck.

We fucked for long moments, stopping every once in a while to keep from coming, wanting to draw it out forever. But I knew that was impossible. I just had to feel what it was like to come in this gorgeous girl.

So I pumped, and slid, and pulled out, and pumped into her again. I kissed her and whispered into her ears about how good she was, and I fucked her harder and harder. When her hands got into my hair and started pulling it, I knew she was going to pop an orgasm. I let her do it. I let her come first, so I could let loose with everything I had.

She groaned and came, flooding my dick with her juices. And I just pumped her harder, ramming it into her, fucking her as hard as I could without tossing us right over the desk and through the gypsum-board wall, into the Computer Science Club office. I pulled out at just the last minute and shot my load right over her head. Jets of come splattered the far wall and sprinkled down over her like sugar.

To this day, my buddies have been wondering what that stain on the wall was all about!

THE GARDENER
Gary Lester

Ann strolled through her garden, gathering roses for her living room. Pedro had just finished pruning a lilac bush when he noticed her coming his way. She smiled and asked him when he thought the bush would produce flowers. The gardener could see her nipples protruding through her light linen blouse. Ann had small, firm breasts and never wore a bra. She must have liked the way her nipples felt when they rubbed against her clothing. He told her she could expect the first round of blooms in a couple of months.

The Southern California sun beat down on them. Ann admired his broad shoulders and muscular physique. Beads of sweat were trickling down his bare tan torso. Ann could smell his masculine musk. She couldn't help herself—she reached over and traced the contours of his thick biceps. Pedro looked up, perplexed at her motion.

Without saying a word, she unbuttoned her blouse and let it drop on the grass. She unzipped her long skirt and pulled it down carefully, stepping over it one foot at a time. Pedro's cock twitched underneath his cotton trousers at the sight of her nakedness.

He cut a Queen Ann's lace and used it to tickle her pink nipples to hardness. With a feathery touch, he trailed the flower down to her crotch. He handed her the flower, grabbed her by the waist, and reached between her legs.

Her pussy was moist and seemed to burn with desire. He spread her lips and tickled her clit. Ann arched her back and stood on her toes, tensing her body. Pedro increased the speed of his finger, bringing Ann to new heights of ecstasy.

He lowered her to the ground carefully and knelt between her legs. With the tip of his tongue, he patted her throbbing clit, pressing harder and harder, making her breathe heavily.

Her opening was dripping with pussy nectar. Pedro was lapping it all up. His cock was painfully hard, ready to penetrate his mistress. He flipped her on her tummy and balancing herself on all fours, priming her downy pussy with his saliva.

He steadied his cock at the base with one hand and aimed it at her eager strawberry patch. Holding her asscheeks apart for easy access, he plunged into her soaking cunt, pushing his cock to the hilt. She let out a high-pitched moan and threw her head back.

Pedro's rhythm increased, occasionally pulling his cock out completely and then thrusting back in forcefully. He held her ass tightly and shoved hard for a few seconds. She could feel his prick wiggling deep inside her cunt. He felt her body tense. Her pussy muscles tightened around his engorged cock. He pumped her hard and fast until she screamed and her body shook with passion. Her pussy contracted, and her fluids dripped down the side of her thigh.

Pedro leaned over her back, his arm around her waist, burying his face into her shoulder blades, and fucked her wildly. He squeezed her body tightly, clenched his ass muscles and pumped. He felt the pressure at the base of his balls building up and moving through the thick, hard shaft. He exploded, shooting streams of steamy thick come into her damp, pulsating cunt. He held his dick inside her until he was completely drained. Then he pulled out.

The two of them collapsed on the lawn staring up at the sunny sky, surrounded by the trees and exotic flowers. He kissed her hand and placed the Queen Ann's lace between her breasts. She closed her eyes and rested her head on his shoulder, thinking about the flower arrangement for her living room.

SISTER-IN-LAW
Tony Gould

Martha was away for the weekend, leaving her husband Roger to spend some time hanging with his buddies. Unfortunately, his buddies had family plans, so Roger was stuck house-sitting.

He had decided to take on some long-forgotten projects when Cynthia barged in, looking to borrow one of Martha's evening gowns for a party. Roger and Cynthia never talked much, and they usually stayed out of each other's way. She never considered him to be one of the brightest men she'd ever met, and he always thought she was kind of snotty.

Cynthia ran upstairs to the bedroom and was raiding her sister's closet when Roger walked in.

"I didn't hear you come in," he said. "What are you up to?"

"I need to borrow a dress for a fund-raiser," she mumbled over her shoulder. "Here's one. I'll try it on. You tell me if it looks good on me."

She started to undress without realizing that her brother-in-law was still in the room. He couldn't believe his eyes. His sister-in-law was standing naked in front of him, trying to squeeze into his wife's dress.

Unlike his wife, Cynthia had huge breasts and a full, round ass. She was voluptuous, but firm. Roger felt his cock harden at the sight of her. He walked over to her and picked up her clothes from the floor. Cynthia started and turned red from embarrassment.

"Oh, my God! I thought you had left the room!" She tried to cover herself with her hands.

Then she noticed his erection pushing against his tight denims, and she gave him a smile. True, he was idiotic, but he was a good-looking, well-built doofus. He was a bit on the rough side, but she was attracted to him nonetheless.

"Well, Roger, do you like what you see?"

"Very much so!" He wore a half-crooked grin.

"So, what are you going to do about it?" she asked. "I haven't got all day!"

He walked over to her, grabbed her by the waist, and pulled her firmly against his body. Staring straight in her eyes, he reached up to her tits and pinched her nipples. Cynthia moaned softly and pushed her cunt against his hard-on. She unzipped his pants freeing his massive cock.

She touched the tip of his cockhead, spreading the

precome around with her thumb. She squeezed the shaft and pushed down and then up several times. Roger picked her up and placed her on the bed. He pinned her hands over her head and covered her mouth with his lips. Their tongues wrestled as they nibbled on each other's lips.

Roger rubbed his prick on her tummy a couple of times and then forced his thick meat into her soaking-wet cunt. She wrapped her legs around his denim-covered legs and pushed her hips up to meet his forceful thrusts.

Roger pushed Cynthia's huge tits together and gobbled on her plump, hard nipples. He licked and nipped at them making her shudder and growl. Suckling on them relentlessly, like a big, dumb, starving baby, he made them swell in his mouth.

Cynthia couldn't bear it any longer. She cupped his head with her hands, holding him down on her sore breasts, and came over and over, crying out with every thrust.

Roger continued feeding on his sister-in-law's tits. Her pussy tightened around his cock. He pumped her harder and faster, until he felt the heaviness building up in his testicles. He was pouncing on her now, maintaining his steady beat until his cock detonated, shooting his fiery liquid into her ravaged cunt.

He pulled out and stroked himself a couple of times. Cynthia jumped up, grabbed his cock, stuffed it in her mouth, and sucked him dry.

After a few moments of deep breathing, he picked up a long red dress and offered it to her.

"This was always my favorite. It'll accentuate your best features," he said and winked at her.

Cynthia took the dress, kissed his cheek, and sprang out of bed.

"I always thought you were sort of an asshole, Roger." She smiled. "A few more sessions like this one, and you're gonna shape up to being the best brother-in-law a girl could ask for!"

BACHELOR PARTY

Jerry Cohen

Alex was feeling a little tipsy, but firmly believed he could take a lot more. He poured his buddies a sixth round of drinks, even as they jumped on the couches and love seats of the hotel suite, as if they were still in elementary school. They were waiting for the girls to arrive, and suffice to say, they were getting impatient.

This was Alex's last time to celebrate before the big day, and he certainly intended to go all out. The crew was getting so raucous, they almost didn't hear the knock on the door. Alex's buddy Sam opened it, and in walked two tall blonde visions.

The guys fell silent quickly. Their mouths dropped, and their eyes followed the girls' every move.

One of the pair placed a tape player on the table and

pressed the play button. Suddenly loud disco music reverberated throughout the suite. They tossed their coats off, exposing their bodies, absolutely nude, save for G-strings, one gold and one metallic red.

The girls started shaking their butts and dancing with each other, moving comfortably around the room. The men were ecstatic. With every twist and shake the men got louder and louder, taking off their shirts and flinging them across the room. Eddie was running around pouring drinks for everyone.

As the dance wound down, Sam took Alex to the bedroom and told him to wait there. Soon enough, the girls danced their way in, closing the door behind them. Both jumped on the bed and pulled Alex down along with them. They started messing with each other's nipples, and wanted the groom-to-be to take a nice, long look before he doomed himself to one lady forever.

They removed their G-strings and started playing with themselves. Poor Alex was sober enough to get an instant erection. He unzipped his pants and pulled out his enormous thick cock. He watched the girls rub their pussies, and he masturbated, despite himself!

Before he knew it, one of the girls made herself comfortable between his legs and sucked his balls into her mouth. She rolled them around gently, tapping them with her tongue. That made Alex's head spin. His cock was oozing with precome. She massaged the liquid around the head and circled the rim with her thumb.

Not wanting to feel left out, the other girl positioned herself next to her girlfriend. She grabbed Alex's shaft and stuffed her mouth with it. Alex was in heaven! His cock and balls were being sucked by two different women, both exquisitely beautiful.

He fell back on the bed, closed his eyes, and let the women work on him. He didn't want to look, he just wanted to feel—and it felt real good. He felt a hand going between his asscheeks to stroke his asshole. The finger pushed its way in, twisting and turning. His dick was rockhard.

He felt two hands rolling his nipples between thumbs and forefingers. The sensations were unbearable. The sucking on his rod became faster and harder. His asshole was being prodded relentlessly, and his balls were floating around in a hot mouth.

He opened his eyes halfway, only to see two blonde heads bobbing up and down, hands searching and probing every crevice of his body. He couldn't hold back any longer. His asshole clenched the finger tightly, his balls tensed inside her mouth, and his cock exploded in the other girl's mouth. His dick was pulled out and he felt two tongues lapping up the hot steamy cream.

They were passing his dick back and forth from mouth to mouth as if it was a gourmet hors d'oeuvre. They licked him clean, leaving not a trace, not a drop to be seen. Then they patted their mouths dry, tucked his dick back into his pants and, without a word, danced their way back into the living room.

Alex was completely fulfilled at his bachelor party. He lay in bed drinking a beer and wondered whether he could get away with having another one.

PERSONAL TRAINER
Joshua Thorpe

Eric was holding Connie's hand making sure that she was lifting the weights properly. She'd been working out for two weeks now, and she was beginning to get the hang of it. She also liked Eric very much.

At first Connie was nervous about being alone in her house with a strange man, but lately she was looking forward to his visits. She tried really hard because she wanted to impress him. And Eric was impressed when he first saw her.

Connie was petite, had full breasts, a tiny waist, and long auburn hair. She had the face of a little girl and the body of a sexy woman. Every time Eric worked with her, he had to try hard not to get an erection.

Today Connie was going out of her way, rubbing up

against him. She loved the way he smelled. When she bent over to lift the next set of weights, Eric felt his cock twitch beneath his spandex shorts. She lay on the bench press with her legs wide open, ready to be spotted.

Eric was standing right behind her, trying not to stare at the tits that looked as if they would spill out of her bodysuit. To his surprise, she reached over her head to where he was standing and grabbed his cock.

"*This* is what I want to lift!" she told him.

His dick popped up instantly. He pulled it over the waistband of his shorts and lowered himself into her mouth. Without asking, he released her large breasts and massaged them, pulling and pinching on her hard nipples.

Connie had taken his cock all the way down her throat, squeezing it tightly between her cheeks. She lifted his balls and stroked the underside of his cock, reaching toward his asshole. When she finally located it, she pushed her finger in gently exploring his insides. Eric was dripping precome into her mouth.

He got up and walked around the front. He removed her work-out clothes, mounted her over the bench press, and guided his cock into her tight, soaking-wet pussy. A loud moan escaped her lips when he stretched her cunt out as he entered.

He pushed deeply inside her and started to pump her full speed. He liked to fuck hard and fast. Connie raised her legs and held them wide apart for him. He grunted with every thrust that he gave her. Connie had never been fucked by someone so powerful before. She arched her back and tilted her hips forward for the full effect of the impact. She came loudly, crying out ecstatically.

Eric steadied himself against the bar of the weights and pumped her forcefully. Beads of sweat trickled down the side of his face and splashed on hers. He felt the pressure build up. With one last hard thrust, he shot his wad deep inside her cunt. He continued to pump until he was completely empty.

Eric got off the bench and sat on the floor besides Connie. A few more sessions like that, and they'd both be in excellent aerobic shape! He wiped himself with his towel and helped her off the bench.

"Okay, Connie, now we're going to work on your gluteus maximus," he said with a half-smile.

HOT SUMMER NIGHT
Ben Torres

The light of the full moon filtered through the filmy clouds of the hot, humid night. The neighborhood guys were hanging out on the street corner, drinking their beer and hungry for action. Most of the townfolk were home keeping cool, their air conditioners working full blast.

Jenny was lying on the grass in her backyard, staring at the sky when Peter, her next-door neighbor, turned the hose on her and doused her with cold water. She was furious, but refreshed.

Her cotton tank top clung to her body, showing off her small breasts and large, hard nipples. Her cutoff denim shorts were dripping water and had become uncomfortably heavy. Peter was chuckling to himself, proud of his achievement. He jumped over the fence and feigned concern. Annoyed, Jenny turned suddenly and slugged him one.

Peter was startled by her response more than he was hurt. He grabbed Jenny and wrestled her to the ground, laughing at her attempt to beat him. Jenny shouted out and complained that she was not amused by any of this. Peter let her go and apologized for his idiotic behavior. Getting what she wanted, Jenny forgave him quickly and offered him a drink.

Together they lay on the grass, staring at the sky. Jenny leaned over and kissed him. Peter responded by kissing her back. Soon they were rolling around their tongues exploring each other's mouths. Lips were being nibbled and chewed. Hands found their way under blouses and skirts.

Jenny managed to get on top of Peter, rocking herself on his erect cock which was fighting to release itself from the denim prison. She unzipped his fly and let the monster loose. It was a thick seven-incher with a head much larger than the shaft.

She held it tight with both hands and squeezed it. A bead of precome oozed out from its hole. Jenny touch the liquid with the tip of her tongue and spread it around. She traced the rim, then under the rim, and moved down the shaft slowly, finding her way to his ballsac.

Peter's cock was painfully hard. He watched her every move, anticipating her next one. She winked and swallowed the beast. She took it all the way down, feeling it push against the back of her throat. Holding it firmly between her lips, she pushed and pulled all the while looking him in the eye.

After she had gotten a good taste of her next-door neighbor, she mounted him. She held his cock at the base and lowered her hot, sweaty cunt on it. Peter closed his eyes and sighed in relief and ecstasy as Jenny's pussy gobbled his meat.

She pounced on him, rocking back and forth every now and then, until her pussy started to contract. She screamed loud enough to alert every one on the block. Her whole body was damp from the heat and from her orgasms.

Peter rolled her over, spread her legs wide, and dove in. She was very happy to get some more cock. He thrust and prodded, making her scream until her throat was getting sore. They didn't care about waking everyone up.

Pete sucked on her nipples while he pumped nonstop. He was licking her all over tasting the saltiness of her sweat. His breathing got heavy. His balls tightened. With a few more hard thrusts, he shot his load into her pussy. He pulled out and let the rest of his come drip on her. He massaged the remainder into her tummy.

Jenny lay on the grass with her legs open, airing out her cunt. Peter collapsed next to her, too tired to utter a word. She got up, got the garden hose, and sprayed him with cold water.

"This'll cool you off!" She laughed at him.

Peter got up and chased her until he caught her.

"Now you're in trouble!" he exclaimed.

He turned her over and gave her butt a couple of slaps.

"As soon as I get my second wind, your ass is mine!"

HALLOWEEN PARTY
Cynthia Freeley

The guests were conversing, laughing, eating, drinking, all in complete disguise. Every year Lou Ann's friends and acquaintances looked forward to her Halloween bashes. She knew how to throw a party.

Unless the guests had arrived with their own partners, they didn't know who anyone else was. No disclosure of identity was one of the rules of the party. Everyone had to be in complete disguise throughout the whole evening.

Lou Ann was dressed as a French Renaissance courtesan. She wore an exquisite powder-blue gown, a wig, and a white contoured mask to hide her face. She mingled among her guests, keeping them in the dark about her identity.

She spotted a woman dressed as a Roman slave girl. She had curly dark hair, held up by gold ribbons, a long white tunic. gold sandals and a golden half-mask. She was tall and walked gracefully. Lou Ann approached her and took her hand.

"Tonight you'll be mine," she told the slave girl.

That was another rule of the party. The guests could "tag" another guest they found desirable to fulfill their hedonistic desires. So long as everyone agreed, anything was acceptable.

The slave girl's "scene" name was Tasha. The two walked around looking for a male to join them. Tasha spotted a man dressed in a nineteenth-century British uniform. He was tall and lean, with dark brown hair. His face was covered with a shiny red mask. The only features painted on the mask were the eyebrows, which gave him an eerie appearance.

The women decided they liked his appearance, so they walked up to him, took his hands, and led him upstairs to one of the bedrooms. Lou Ann closed the doors behind them and dimmed the lights. Tasha removed her tunic, but kept her gold sandals and slave bracelets. Lou Ann removed only the gown, but left on her pantaloons and bodice. The soldier did not remove any of his clothing. They all had to keep their masks on.

The three of them lay on the king-sized water bed and began to grope one another. Tasha reached out for Lou Ann's tits and lifted them over the bodice. She then grabbed her nipples and rolled them around between her thumbs and forefingers. After they were good and hard, she took each one in her mouth and sucked on them, making them swell even more.

The soldier spread Tasha's legs and lapped up her juices. He stimulated her clit with long, slow strokes of his tongue. He inserted two fingers into her dripping cunt and rotated them while thrusting in and out. Tasha was shuddering and moaning, all the while continuing to suck and nibble on Lou Ann's precious nipples.

Lou Ann's pussy was throbbing. She unbuttoned the flap of her pantaloons and masturbated herself. The soldier's cock was becoming impatient, struggling to free itself and invade new territory. He stopped eating Tasha's cunt, rose and undid his pants. He pulled out a huge chunk of uncut meat that was standing at attention. He stroked the shaft, pulling back the foreskin and exposing a fat purple head that was glistening with precome.

At the sight of this monstrosity, the girls giggled, licked their lips and jumped at it immediately. With the tips of their tongues, they tickled the head and the hole, licking the precome. They circled his rim and continued down the shaft, moving on to his balls. Lou Ann sucked on each fleshy sphere. Tasha nibbled and pulled on his foreskin while stroking his cockhead with her thumb.

The soldier took control of his cock and pierced Tasha with it. She let out short bursts of breath with each invading thrust. Lou Ann positioned herself over Tasha's head and lowered her pussy for the slave girl to feast on. Tasha encompassed Lou Ann's cunt with her lips and delicately thrust her tongue into the hot, wet opening.

Lou Ann and the soldier were French-kissing while Tasha was being fucked. Lou Ann pinched and twisted the soldier's nipples, and he returned the favor. The three of them were humping and gyrating in unifying rhythm, while being completely unaware of each others' identities.

Tasha's cunt was being ravaged by the soldier's prick. His thrusts were becoming increasingly harder. Lou Ann's nipples were becoming sore from the soldier's relentless pinching and pulling but he had no intention of stopping. Her pussy was throbbing from Tasha's probing tongue. Lou Ann's body stiffened. With a loud moan that was absorbed into the soldier's mouth, Lou Ann came, her fluids dripping directly into Tasha's mouth.

At the taste of Lou Ann's excited pussy Tasha began to climax. The soldier focused his attention on Tasha's nipples, heightening the intensity of her orgasm. Her pussy contracted forcefully, creating extra pressure around the soldier's cock. Lou Ann had moved behind the soldier and was rimming his asshole with her tongue.

The soldier leaned over Tasha, held her down by her wrists, and pummeled her pulsating cunt mercilessly. Lou Ann's tenacious tongue did not skip a beat. His asshole was covered with her spit. The combination of sensations was more than enough for him. With one last hard thrust, he shot his cannon, spilling his creamy liquid into her quivering cunt.

They fell into each other's arms and rested for a

while. Later, they got dressed, the soldier bowed and kissed the ladies' hands, thanking them for their hospitality, and escorted them back to the main hall. They mingled in the crowd and continued to search for new fuck partners to occupy themselves for the rest of the night.

LIMO RIDE
Jamie Christiansen

The stretch limo waited on the busy New York City street, parked by the water hydrant. Jackie came out of her brownstone apartment building wearing a long, form-fitting silver dress. The shiny satin fabric reflected the street and car lights, giving her a celestial glow.

She was tall and slender. Her golden hair was pinned up loosely in a bun. Her breasts were firm and round, featuring long nipples that pointed toward the sky. Her skin was silky smooth, her eyes deep blue, and her lips a burgundy red.

She scurried to the limo, her breasts slightly jiggled with her every move. The chauffeur opened the door for her and she slid into the backseat. Ken greeted her with a kiss on her cheek and a glass of champagne. He was taking her to the opera.

He lifted her hand and placed a kiss on each of her fingers. Then he placed one in his mouth deliberately and sucked gently on it. Turning her hand, he placed a light kiss at the base of her wrist. He grinned and moved closer so that he could nibble at her earlobe. She shivered a bit, even though it wasn't cold. He nibbled his way down her neck to where her breasts parted.

Jackie lifted his head and met his lips in a deep, probing kiss. Their tongues met and grappled, her fingers moving through his hair. Using his body weight, Ken pushed her gently down the leather seat and ran his hands up and down her body.

She moaned back in his mouth, and he down pulled her satin dress. His mouth was on her nipples, sucking them, licking around the aureoles. She was breathing hard through her nose. The leather seats creaked. The chauffeur was focused on the road, but occasionally stole a glimpse at the horny couple.

Ken felt himself getting hard and pushed his hips gently into hers. She unbuckled his belt and grasped his immense hard-on. Squeezing firmly, she stroked his cock a few times and then took it in her mouth. She opened her throat and swallowed it, twirling her tongue around the shaft and sucking it hard. She nosed around his balls, took one then the other into her mouth, and rolled them around gently, directing them with her skilled tongue. She could tell he was on the verge of exploding. She pulled her dress over her hips, leaned back, and opened herself to him.

"Fuck me, Ken," she whispered.

His dick had been well lubricated by the combination of her saliva and precome. She shifted to give him easier access, one long leg resting on the back of the front seat and the other over his shoulder. Holding on to his rock-hard cock, he eased into her tight, wet hole. He felt her shudder beneath him. Then, she placed her hands on his hips and pulled him closer, holding him with her legs.

He started moving—slowly at first, then faster and faster until he was slamming in and out of her so rapidly that he was knocking the wind out of her. She threw her hands over her head and closed her eyes. His every shove evoked a breathy moan from her lips.

Finally she couldn't take any more and came with a harsh cry. As he saw her face contort with her climax, he felt the tightening of his own balls, followed by a cascade of come which filled her tight passage. As the final spasm passed, he collapsed against her.

After a couple of minutes, Ken helped Jackie put her dress back on. She combed her hair and applied fresh lipstick. He adjusted himself, even as the limo pulled up outside the theater. The chauffeur opened the doors for them, and Ken took Jackie's hand to help her out of the car. Ken gave her a smile and a wink, and escorted her to the opera.

THE TEASE
Claire Watson

Lisa pranced around the living room barefoot, wearing her tiny terry-cloth shorts and her skintight tank top. Her brother's friend Brian was watching her every move, feeling his cock growing under his denims.

Lisa enjoyed teasing her brother's friends. It gave her a thrill knowing that they got blue balls. She was holding an ice-cold bottle of soda pop and was gulping it down suggestively as she stared at him. Brian was horny and nervous.

She sat next to him on the sofa and leaned back on the armrest. She placed one leg on the floor and rested the other on the back of the sofa, giving Brian a clear view of her crotch. Her tight shorts accentuated the slit of her pussy.

She finished the soda pop and positioned the bottle between her tender fleshy thighs. She continued staring at him while tracing her lips with her index finger.

"Hey, Brian, it may be a while before my brother returns from the gym. Didn't you know that he was going to be there tonight?"

"Uh...yeah, but he said he'd be back by now," he answered, his voice cracking.

"So are you just going to sit there like a lump waiting for him?"

"What do you mean?" he asked, embarrassed.

She didn't answer him. She gave him a devilish grin and subtly moved her hands to her breasts. She ran her fingers over her hardened nipples and opened her legs even wider. The shifting of her position made the bottle tilt into the slit of her cunt.

Brian cleared his throat and licked his lips. He was at a total loss. Lisa grabbed the bottle and pressed it against her pussy, rubbing it up and down her slit. Her breathing got louder. Her eyes glazed. She was getting wet watching Brian become more nervous by the minute.

"I bet you'd like to fuck me!" she announced.

"I'd love to fuck you, Lisa," he answered earnestly.

"Well, I'm not going to let you, Brian," she replied cruelly.

She pulled her tank top over her head, exposing her large, round tits. Her tiny nipples were like baby rosebuds waiting to bloom. She lifted one tit to her lips and began sucking on it, never taking her gaze from his. She slipped her hands down her shorts and fingered her damp hole, sighing from the pleasure she was giving herself.

Brian was rubbing the bulge between his legs.

"Pull your dick out, Brian, and jerk it. I want to see how big it can get."

Having gotten permission, he unzipped his fly and pulled out his erection. To her surprise, his prick was huge. It was long and wide, with a large purple-red head that looked like a helmet. Her eyes widened at the sight.

"Wow! I never thought that such a scrawny guy like you would have such a big dick! I'm impressed."

"Thanks," he answered, proud of his asset. He thought better of complaining about her saying he was scrawny.

"I wanna sit on it, Brian."

He moved to the middle of the sofa. Lisa removed her clothes and straddled Brian, with her back toward him. He held onto her hips as she squatted down on his massive hard-on. He angled his cock to meet her hole. She took it slowly, feeling the walls of her cunt stretch to new limits.

Her cunt swallowed his whole cock. He took in a deep breath relishing the feel of her wet, hot, tight cunt. Once her pussy adjusted to its thickness, she began to push herself up and down. He stretched his long legs forward and leaned back, holding onto her, helping her keep her balance. He watched the crack of her ass open wide as she pounced on him.

She was grunting like a wild animal, increasing her

speed. She pulled his dick out and put it back in, resuming her rhythm. Brian thrust his hips up in order to increase the impact of her pussy slamming against him.

She arched her back, closed her eyes, and massaged her clit until she came. She let out a loud scream and fell backward on Brian. Her heart was pounding, and she was gasping.

Brian wasn't done yet. He was going to make her pay for torturing and humiliating him. He placed her on her back on the couch, lifted her legs over his shoulders, and pushed his way into her tight asshole. He shoved his cock all the way in without any lubrication. Lisa screamed, this time from pain.

Brian fucked her asshole raw, stretching it with every deep thrust. He pushed her tits together and took both her nipples into his mouth. He sucked hard on them, biting and pulling, making them swell. Lisa's pain slowly turned into pleasure.

Finally Brian felt the pressure built up deep within his sack. He pummeled her a few more times, his balls slapping her meaty cheeks. He exploded, spilling his come in spurts. He pulled his cock out and shoved it in her mouth, forcing her to take it down her throat.

She cleaned him up, swallowing every last drop of his cream. He pulled his dick out, winked at her, and patted her on the head.

"Good job, Lisa. I always told your brother you were a hot piece of ass!"

He got up, dressed, and walked out, knowing that she was completely satisfied and somewhat humiliated.

LONG LEGS, SILK STOCKINGS

Jack Tobie

The alarm went off. Ryan groaned and dragged himself out of bed. After picking out his clothes for work, he went into the bathroom to take a shower. His girlfriend Megan was already in there, having gotten up earlier.

She was resting one leg on the toilet seat, pulling up her silk stockings and attaching them to her garter belt. She looked up and winked at Ryan. Her legs were endless. Ryan thought how she had the most beautiful thighs, and the stockings only served to accentuate them.

She slipped into her black patent-leather shoes and left the bathroom. All she was wearing were her stockings, her black lace panties, and a matching bra. Ryan enjoyed watching the slight jiggle of her butt as she scurried around the apartment.

Ryan forgot all about his shower. He approached Megan from behind, put his hands around her waist, and nibbled on the edge of her ear. He liked the way her hair smelled. Megan leaned into him and rubbed her behind up against his hardening cock.

Ryan cupped her breasts and squeezed gently. He felt her nipples pushing into his palms. He bent her over the bed and groped her ass. He kneeled behind her and stroked her long legs. He kissed her calves, the back of her knees, the inside of her thighs.

He pushed her legs farther apart and slipped her panty crotch over to one side. With the tip of his tongue, he licked her clit and prodded her damp pussy-hole. Megan wiggled her ass in his face and moaned.

Holding on to her long legs, Ryan continued to lap her wet cunt. His cock was painfully hard. He was rubbing it up against her leg, feeling the texture of her silk stocking. He got up and tapped the head of his cock against her clit. Megan shuddered at his touch.

He held his dick at an angle and pushed the head halfway into her hole. He immediately pulled out and pushed in again. He teased her like this a couple of times, and then he plunged his prick deep inside her soaking cunt.

Holding onto her hips, he shoved hard into her, making her growl like an animal. She was standing on her toes to give him better access to her cunt. Ryan grabbed her hair and tugged it slightly backward with each thrust forward.

Megan screamed wildly and climaxed strongly, pushing back against his pounding hips. Ryan leaned forward, slipped his hands under her breasts, and rolled her nipples between his thumbs and forefingers. He nibbled on her back and shoulders as he pumped her hard and fast.

He pulled her hair over to one side and chewed on her earlobe. The sensation of her pulsating cunt and his body rubbing on hers was too much for him. He stuck his tongue inside her ear and whispered to her that he was about to come.

He pounced on her a couple of times, pulled his cock out, and shot streams of hot milky come all over her legs. With his cock, he massaged his liquid up and down her thighs and all the way down to her ankles. Her silk stockings clung to her skin, sticky with his cream.

Then Ryan licked his fluids off her legs, nibbling at her flesh as he was cleaning her up. Megan was breathless from the experience. Suddenly they realized they were late for work. They panicked, but then decided to call in sick, take the rest of the day off, and continue fucking.

BLIND DATE
Fred Richards

Steve and Sandy met for the first time in the back of their friends' car, on their way to a drive-in movie. Both were nervous about meeting each other this way, but were also pleasantly surprised when it finally happened.

Steve was not very tall, but he was lean and muscular. He had short dark brown hair, dark brown eyes, and a bright smile. Sandy was petite, with full, round breasts, shoulder-length red hair, and hazel eyes. They were attracted to one another instantly.

After the movie was over they went back to their friends' house. Their friends disappeared conveniently into the bedroom, leaving the two of them alone. Steve and Sandy were happy to have some time to themselves.

After some light conversation, Steve leaned over and

kissed Sandy. Her lips tasted sweet and her tongue danced around with his. He nibbled on her neck, and she breathed more heavily. She ran her fingers down his back, bringing them around the front of his torso. She traced the contours of his muscled belly and scraped her nails over his nipples.

Steve's cock shifted in his pants. He felt it grow and harden. He pressed his bulge against her crotch. He could feel the heat between her legs. He slipped a hand under her mini-dress and ran a finger up the slit of her pussy. Sandy shuddered at his touch. He stroked her a few times until he felt her moisture seeping through her cotton panties.

She found the waistband of his jeans, unbuttoned it, and moved her small hand to locate the head of his cock. It was wet with precome. She rubbed the head with her thumb in circles, spreading the liquid all around. Steve thought he would explode from the sensation.

He pulled off her panties. Sandy responded to his every move. She unzipped his fly and freed his imposing rod. She held it with her tiny hands and kneaded it, pushing down and pulling up as hard as she could.

Steve's heart was pounding. Sandy directed his cock into her tiny wet hole. He pushed the head in slowly. Sandy moaned as her tight pussy stretched to accommodate the massive intruder.

He shoved his prick in to the hilt, held it in place for a couple of seconds, relishing the hot, wet, tight feel, and then began to pound away. Sandy was almost whimpering from the intense pleasure. Her pussy had never been stretched so widely or probed so deeply. She came instantly, her fluids oozing down her cunt each time Steve pulled out his shaft.

Her burning, pulsating pussy massaged Steve's cock. He grabbed onto her head and came violently, his cock-head bursting with explosive spurts of come. He pummeled her until his meat was fully drained. He kept it inside her until it began to soften. Then he pulled out of her throbbing, sore pussy.

They kissed passionately for a while. After they got themselves together, they exchanged phone numbers and made plans to meet again without the company of their friends. They both agreed that this was the only successful blind date they had ever had.

WINE TASTING
Philip Woll

Recently I received an invitation to a private wine tasting. I had no great knowledge of wines, but decided to go anyway. To me, if a wine tasted okay, I drank it. I didn't like anything too dry or too sweet. I knew that red wine went well with red meat, and white was good with seafood. I had no idea what rosé was all about, and frankly, I didn't care.

The gathering was at a loft downtown. The guests were mingling, tasting the various brands that were displayed on one long buffet table. To my disgust, they were sipping and spitting. I never expected to see such classy-looking folk behave that way, but I guess it was part of the judging. I just wanted to meet some broads and get a few free drinks.

A great-looking chick approached me, handed me a glass of red, and asked me to savor the bouquet. I had no fuckin' idea what she was talking about. However, she had a great pair of tits, and a knockout bod. I told her I'd rather savor *her* bouquet.

To my surprise she didn't slap me. She smiled at me and told me to follow her, which I did, of course. She led me into a bedroom, locked the door behind me, and proceeded to strip off her clothes. I couldn't believe my eyes.

There she was, completely naked in front of me. Her hooters were huge, with long, thick nipples pointing upward. I began to salivate like a hungry dog. Her pussy had a patch of hair on her mound, but her labia were clean shaven. I could see the tip of her clit peeking through her lips.

She lay on the bed, spread her long legs as wide apart as she could, and she poured the glass of wine on her tummy. The red liquid trickled down her snatch, changing the color of her pink pussy to a light red.

"Come and savor my bouquet," she told me, smiling and sipping what was left in the glass.

I jumped at the offer. I dove into her hotbox and lapped up the wine. The smell of the alcohol mixed with her musky aroma, making my head spin. This was a fine blend. I licked her clit, pushing down on it with the rough part of my tongue and flicking it sideways.

Her legs shook and she growled, rocking her hips up and down. Her pussyhole dripped her own fluids, which I sucked in with relish. She had become my personal bottle of fine wine, but I had no intention of spitting out her juice. I probed her hole with my tongue and circled around it.

My dick was hurting. It was dancing and twitching under my pants. I unzipped my fly quickly and removed my slacks. I got on the bed and told her it was time to taste my concoction. I grabbed the back of her head and shoved my massive member in her mouth, pushing it down her throat.

She gagged at first, but then she relaxed and her throat expanded, taking me in smoothly. I held her head firmly, fucking it in slow, rhythmic motions. Her moans of pleasure were muffled by my thick prick.

She rubbed her clit fast and furious with one hand while her other hand was busy exploring my asshole. She circled my hole with the fleshy part of her index finger and then pushed it as far as it would go. She pressed down firmly and twirled around, making me crazy with excitement.

She climaxed strongly, her body jerking violently, trying to scream with her mouth full. I didn't let go of her head. I continued to fuck it, increasing my speed. Her finger tortured my asshole relentlessly.

I couldn't stand it anymore. My balls felt like they weighed a ton. The pressure in my sac was unbearable. I held her steady and thrust deep down, smashing my testicles against her chin. I exploded all over her mouth, flooding her with my hot, creamy come.

The liquid flowed down the side of her mouth. Each time I pushed in, more come oozed out. She swallowed with each new spurt. She licked under my balls and around her lips and chin—whatever she could reach with her tongue. She gulped it down, sucking me hard, trying to extract more.

She was completely satiated. Her eyes were glazed and her belly was full. She told me that I cleaned out her palate and she was ready for more wine tasting. She asked me to hang around because she'd have to cleanse again after a few more sips. I obliged gladly.

If I only knew what wine tasting was all about, I would have majored in it. Now I plan to attend every event and become an expert. I will be a top-notch palate cleanser!

PONY RIDE
Jamie Christiansen

Scott was brushing down his pony's shiny coat lovingly. It was a slow-paced day at the ranch. Most of the regulars were seeking shelter from the sweltering heat in their homes. Scott took the opportunity to groom his animal and go for a ride.

Vicky strolled in, looking for a suitable horse. She wanted to go for a ride, too. She noticed Scott sitting on a stool, buffing his pony's hooves, and walked over to greet him. He looked up as she was approaching and saw her long bare legs, her tight shorts cutting into her crotch, and her clingy cotton blouse accentuating her perky breasts.

Scott had been lusting after Vicky ever since he first met her. She squatted down next to him and blew him a kiss. He noticed the fullness of her cleavage and felt his dick twitch. She was talking to him, but he found it hard to concentrate on her words.

He leaned over and kissed her cheek. Vicky gave him a kiss back. Suddenly they embraced and rolled on the ground, groping and rubbing their bodies together. Scott kicked the stall door shut for more privacy.

He tore her blouse open and attacked her tits. He held them together and nuzzled her hard pink nipples, licking around the aureoles. Vicky was breathing heavily grinding her crotch against his growing bulge.

He pulled down her shorts, exposing her moist pussy. He removed his pants quickly and jumped on her. Her cunt was burning. He stroked his prick between the lips of her pussy, pressing down hard for more friction.

He tongued her mouth once again and simultaneously inserted his cock into her hungry pussy. Vicky wrapped her legs around his and pushed up her hips to meet his every thrust. She was moaning into his mouth, her nostrils flaring as her breath escaped her lungs.

The smell of their musk mixed with the odor of the pony, and the stable was intoxicating. Scott pulled his dick out and flipped her over on all fours. He parted her asscheeks and reentered her throbbing vagina. He pushed into her asshole with his thumb, making her tremble.

Vicky played with her clit until she climaxed, her body jerking backward, slamming into Scott's hips. He pumped her, grunting with each thrust. His cock was swimming in her juices. His balls tightened and released an explosion of come into her pulsating hole.

He pulled out and wiped his cock into the crack of her ass. He turned her over and kissed her, holding her tightly in his arms. They got dressed, saddled their ponies, and went for a ride. They didn't exchange any more words, but they had a newfound understanding of each other.

THE CANDY STORE
Philip Woll

She walked into the store just as I was getting ready to close down. I waited patiently for her to make her purchase so that I could go home but she was taking her sweet time.

I thought I should tell her I was closed, but my heart wasn't in it. I watched her as she looked at every row of candies and chocolates. She was beautiful. Her curly light brown bangs were falling in her eyes. Her lips were full and tender.

She was wearing a tiny low-cut cotton top that ended right under her full breasts. Her shorts were high cut, sunk between each round, firm buttcheek. She picked a cherry-flavored lollipop. I wondered how many of her licks it would take to reach the chewy center.

She paid me for it and leaned on the counter, sucking on her pop, staring at me.

"Is there anything else you'd like?" I asked her.

"I'd like to suck on something else." She winked at me.

I realized she was craving for meat, not candy. I locked the door and pulled down the vinyl shade. I stood in front of her and unzipped my fly. She knelt down and took my member into her sweetened mouth, right beside her lollipop.

"Mmmm, this is very tasty. It's my favorite kind of candy!" she teased.

Starting at the base, she used the tip of her tongue to lick my hardened cock. She swirled her tongue around, licking first on top, then on the bottom of the shaft. Taking my dick fully into her mouth, she applied pressure to the shaft. The little point of her tongue skimmed around the head and circled the rim. I braced my hands against her shoulders as she licked her way back down toward my balls.

She was salivating cherry spit all over me. She traced my balls with her lollipop, making them sticky and sweet.

"Candy-coated balls are my favorite!" She winked at me.

She took one into her mouth and began to suck off the sticky coating. She rolled one of the sacs around in her mouth, using the raspy part of her tongue to get every drop. She held on to my stiff shaft with both her hands and pushed and pulled firmly. She was milking it thoroughly.

My fingers clenched in her hair as I felt the pressure

coming from somewhere under her tongue. I pulled my cock out of her mouth and erupted in a rush of come, leaving a string of pearly beads on her cleavage. She wiped a few drops off with her lollipop, then licked it off.

"It didn't take me too long to get to the chewy center," she said proudly.

I helped her get back on her feet, and she helped me lock up the store for the night. Every night my girlfriend dropped by to pick me up, but not before she sucked me off, using some sweet from the store.

"Tomorrow it's going to be vanilla-fudge-swirl ice cream!" she announced as we drove off.

THE BOOB TUBE
Gary Benderfield

We sat on the couch, watching mindless television shows. Julia was my next-door neighbor. We hung out almost every night after work, trying to relax together after work. We liked the same sitcoms and other shows. We'd pour ourselves a couple of drinks and gossip about the other neighbors.

Tonight we were just plain bored. Julia said that a coworker had lent her an adult video. She asked if I'd be interested in watching it with her. We agreed to watch it together, and the minute one of us felt uncomfortable, we'd turn it off.

She popped the tape into the machine. Larger-than-life cocks were aiming at the camera and getting sucked off by women with heavy makeup, excessive jewelry, and big hairdos. We were both turned on! We liked every cheesy scene, no matter how vulgar it seemed.

"Hey, let's pretend we're the actors!" she said enthusiastically.

I looked at her, wondering if she was being sarcastic.

"Okay, I'll be the guy with the huge dick, and you can be the slut who sucks me off!" I replied, intentionally sarcastic.

Little did I know that she was serious and didn't pick up on my sarcasm. She got up and removed all her clothing seductively. She danced around the living room and stopped in front of me.

My dick had a mind of its own. As much as I was shocked by her behavior and was trying to think of her as my buddy, my cock thought otherwise. It was stiff as a board, and it was trying to escape.

Licking her lips, she kneeled in front of me. She unzipped me and released the eager monster. She grabbed my shaft from the base and tapped her lips with the head. She parted them and inhaled my meat, sucking hard. She nibbled and suckled down the side of my prick, staring straight into my eyes all along.

I didn't know how talented Julia was. Her performance was better than the actress in the X-rated movie. She pulled each one of my balls in her mouth and rolled them around. She licked under my sac and moved up to the shaft, concentrating on the head. Just when I thought I would explode, she stopped blowing me.

"Fuck me, baby! Stick your hard cock in my pussy and give it to me hard!"

That was the best line I ever heard. I made a mental note to ask for her autograph after the show was over. She was on all fours, her ass wiggling in my face. I licked my fingers and shoved two of them up her hot little snatch.

She was tight and wet. Her pussy was burning. She moaned loudly as I twisted, turned, and shook my fingers inside her. Her juices were flowing heavily. I held onto my manhood and poked her slash. I dove as deep as I could, pounding her hard and fast. She grunted and moaned each time I pummeled her pussy.

She screamed and cried, calling me all kinds of names. I slapped her ass for being a foulmouthed bitch, and with that she exploded. Her orgasms came one after another. Her body shook wildly, lifting off the floor.

Her muscle contractions were so powerful that my dick felt as if it was in a strong vacuum. I dug into her fleshy cheeks and fucked her pussy raw. I shot my load filling her cunt with what seemed like a quart of gooey come. My creamy liquid oozed out of her hole, down her soft thighs.

I pulled out, and she turned around quickly and took my milky prick into her mouth. Unlike the actresses in the video, she sucked me off swallowing every drop. She was fantastic! We clicked off the movie and contemplated our performance.

We decided to act out a different role every night from then on. We even played around with the idea of making our own movies. Stars were in our eyes and heat between our legs. Our pastime had altered, and we were happier for it!

THE BABY-SITTER
T. Grant

I returned home earlier than expected from my date, which didn't work out very well. Being a single father isn't easy, especially when it comes to dating.

The house was dark. Tanya had probably put the baby to sleep by now. I walked up the stairs to the bedrooms. I peeked into the baby's room. He was fast asleep. I walked over to the guest bedroom. The door was slightly ajar.

I looked for Tanya. To my surprise, she had one hand up her dress and was playing with herself. I wasn't sure what I should do. I cleared my throat and tapped on the door.

"Tanya, are you in there?" I called out.

"Oh, Mr. Taylor, you're home!" she responded in a startled voice.

"Yes, my date wasn't very successful." I pushed the door open and walked in.

"And how was your evening with little Jeremy?"

"He's a doll, Mr. Taylor. You have the most beautiful baby. Never gives me a hard time." The tension eased off her face.

"I'm really sorry to hear about your date," she said earnestly.

"It's not easy finding a woman who's willing to start a relationship with a man who already has a child." I answered.

"Well, they have no idea what they're missing. You're a great guy. You're sweet, gentle, and very handsome."

I was flattered by her comments and for the first time started wondering what it would be like to be with her. She was still in college working part-time to earn a little extra cash. She was a gorgeous gal. She had a small physique, a soft, round face, long, fine hair, and large baby-blue eyes. She looked a lot younger than she was.

"That's very sweet of you, Tanya. I wish I could find someone who would appreciate me the way you do!"

"What's wrong with me, Mr. Taylor?"

I was stunned at how forward she was. This was an unbelievable opportunity for me.

"Nothing at all. You're perfect, but don't you think I'm a little old for you?"

"I don't care about that. Besides, most guys my age are still immature. I find you a lot more interesting and attractive."

She walked toward me, stood on her tiptoes, and put

her arms around my neck, giving me a peck on the lips. I embraced her tiny waist, pulled her against my body, and returned the kiss. I parted her lips with the tip of my tongue and explored her mouth. She met my tongue with hers and repeated the moves, twirling her tongue around mine.

I felt my cock harden. She must have felt it, too, because she gave a little moan and pressed her mound against my bulge. I carried her over to the guest bed and placed her down carefully. I sat next to her and continued to kiss her.

She placed her hand on my covered erection and stroked it through my pants. She found the zipper and opened it slowly. Her small hand took hold of my pulsing muscle and pulled it out gently. Her fingers fluttered softly up and down my aching cock.

Slipping my hand under her short linen dress, I stroked the insides of her silky thighs. She shuddered at my touch and parted her legs. My hand inched its way up until my fingers located the band of her panties. I slid a finger under and touched the moist lips of her pussy lightly.

Tanya growled softly into my mouth and pressed harder against me. I traced the outline of her slit and spread the wetness up and down her crack with my fingers. Tanya was trembling in my arms, her breath quickening, and her tongue wrestling with mine more frantically.

With both hands, I eased her panties down her slim thighs and over her knees. They dropped to her ankles. Without breaking the kiss, she tossed them off. Still attached at the lips, I removed my shirt. With her help, my pants came off.

I sat back on the bed, my massive hard-on reaching up toward the ceiling. Her tiny fingers caressed my quivering cock, and she pushed and pulled with both hands. My head was spinning, and my heart was beating painfully hard.

Tanya leaned back on the bed and opened her legs wide for me. The plump vaginal lips parted with the spreading of her legs, exposing a glistening hard nub. I mounted her and lowered myself, holding my dick at the base of the shaft for guidance. I touched the tip of her clitoris with the head of my cock and pressed against it.

Tanya raised her hips, hungry for more. I stroked her clit a couple of times and slid my rigid cock down her wet opening. Her hands clenched at her sides, and she was staring into my eyes with anticipation. I pushed the head in, and she sighed with contentment.

I continued to push very slowly, and her cunt swallowed my steel pole bit by bit. Gripping her asscheeks, I pulled her body against mine and thrust my prick deep inside her. Tanya wrapped her legs around my thighs and held me firmly, her hands sliding up my back.

I began to pump her vigorously, increasing the speed of my thrusts, driving my cock relentlessly into her tight cunt. The burning heat and wetness of her pussy brought me to a state of mindless ecstasy. Her growls and grunts were getting louder and louder. Her body jerked forward, and the juices flowed out of her cunt, soaking my swollen meat.

I shoved my cock as deep as I could, feeling the sperm boiling in the depths of my balls. The pressure built to a peak and rushed out in a violent explosion, sending my steamy come up her contracting cunt. I drove into her a couple of more times and pulled out, collapsing next to her soft, tender body.

We lay in each other's arms all night, dozing, waking, groping one another, and dozing again. Since then, she's been coming over every afternoon. Our relationship has evolved beyond baby-sitter/employer, and I've stopped searching for the perfect mate!

ON THE BALCONY
Severin Waileha

She was the sexiest girl I'd ever seen. God knew what one summer could do to a nineteen-year-old girl. Her hair was fluffy and sunlit, her eyes sparkling. Her smile was white and perfect.

We'd been messing around in the kitchen, I'd sprayed her with a nozzle until she was soaked. We'd stumbled out onto the balcony and tumbled down on the tanning chairs. She was braless, and her T-shirt clung to her like a second skin. The nipples on her ripe, round breasts had hardened through the wet fabric. Her faded jeans dried slowly—I couldn't believe how tightly they fit her. They were little girls' cutoff jeans, and there was definitely a woman's body in them. The denim edges around her thighs were pressing into her skin under the damp fringe. I stared at the button and licked my lips, waiting for it to simply pop open.

Lying there in the sun, she looked so fuckable that I had to get closer. I moved in for the kill, slipping my hands between us, tickling her. She threw her head back and laughed like crazy, grabbing for my hands, wriggling that pert body of hers. I kept at it, and she screamed my name. I could feel her ribs and the tight flesh of her belly through her T-shirt. She felt so full and ripe in my hands that I had to stop, for fear that I would come in my pants.

She grabbed my wrists and pinned them over my head, straddling me and grinning mischievously. She must have felt the bulge of my cock between her legs. She had to know how badly I wanted her.

We calmed down slowly, but her smile just broadened. She leaned over and put her lips on mine. We started making out there on the balcony, in the summer breeze, with my arms folded over my head and my cock throbbing like thunder beneath her crotch.

I peeled her T-shirt out of her jeans and popped open the denim. I pulled those tiny shorts down around her thighs, and we giggled at how tight they were. Pulling away her creamed-up silk panties, I slowly, exquisitely pushed my thick young cock into her wet vagina. We gasped and laughed. I couldn't believe how good it felt. This pretty, sexy, gorgeous girl was mine. And she was riding me, and I was pumping away.

Those pussylips of hers sucked my penis royally. She leaned forward and dug her nails into my chest as she pulled her ass high in the air and pumped it down again and again. My cock went so slick that I would have fallen out if she hadn't been so fantastically tight.

I slid my fingers up under the hem of that tight, wet T-shirt of hers and felt her moist titties. There were so soft and firm, titties that I'd seen poking through a dozen T-shirts all summer. Feeling those nipples between my fingers—feeling my big cock plunging in that young pussy—it was enough to send me into orbit!

When I started to come, I unleashed my secret weapon. I began pumping my hips up into her, giving her a ride like those little horsie machines in front of candy stores. She was on top, in control. She moved herself forward, laughing and giggling, then moaning. We came together, yelling and screaming at the top of our lungs, right out there on the balcony for the whole wide world to see. When she started coming, it felt as if her pussy was sucking my heart out through my cock! My come flew into her at a thousand miles an hour.

She collapsed on me, and we kissed and cuddled. She fell asleep on me, and I caught a few winks myself.

I couldn't help it, though. A half-hour later, she woke up with my dick hard inside her pussy again!

HOLIDAY GIFT
Nicholas White

Wearing only a red satin ribbon wrapped all around her body, Nelly danced wildly for her boyfriend Joel. She was grinding her hips and swirling her hands to jolly holiday tunes. It was Christmas Eve, and she would have just about done anything to please her handsome sweetheart.

Joel was sitting naked on the couch, a little tipsy from the spiked eggnog, stroking his enormous, thick prick. Nelly's bouncing breasts had given him a hard-on. Squatting in front of him, she played with her nipples, plumping them with her fingertips, and tickling them with her polished nails. Then she got up and twirled around, landing on his lap.

Joel gave his girl a kiss. He cupped her breasts and

squeezed gently, lowering his lips to her nipple. He
sucked it into his mouth, flicked his tongue around it
and released it then going for the other. Her nipples
were becoming swollen and red, but he couldn't help
himself. He worked her tits just a bit longer.

Tracing his way down her toned tummy, he tickled
her belly button, and continued till he reached her high
mound. He pinched the flesh, making her squirm and
moan. With two fingers, he parted her pussylips and
stroked her protruding clit. Nelly was breathing heavily,
pushing her hips toward his stroking finger.

Joel's cock was aching for some action. She turned to
face him. Grabbing his meat with both her hands, she
massaged it between her palms. The firm, hot friction
made his cock ooze a few droplets of precome, and he
couldn't help letting out a soft moan. Nelly lowered her
head to his cock and sipped the salty fluid. She closed
her lips around the thick glistening head, and slowly
sucked the shaft deep into her mouth, inch by inch.

Joel was groaning now, almost trying to pull away
from Nelly's oral caresses. When she felt his dick was
thoroughly lubricated, Nelly spread her pussylips to
expose her opening for his pulsing muscle. She lowered
herself onto his cock, stopping to take a deep breath
after the head had been absorbed into her velvety cunt.
With a sudden thrust of his hips, Joel drove the shaft as
far in as it would go.

Nelly shuddered and growled as her pussy stretched
to accommodate his massive penis. He flicked his
thumbs over her hard red nipples, forcing her to buck

and shift. She bounced on him, increasing her tempo, her pussy ever-tightening around his cock. Involuntary grunts escaped from her mouth as her body tensed and spasmed. She was having orgasm after orgasm.

Joel gripped the firm cheeks of her ass and pulled her body down. He pushed and pulled her body, up and down his steel pole, each time thrusting his throbbing cock farther into her cunt. Nelly squeezed his nipples gently while licking his neck.

Joel couldn't hold back anymore. The boiling pressure in the depths of his balls exploded into jets of steamy thick come, shooting into her burning, wet cunt.

Joel's body went limp. Sweat trickling down the sides of his face. Nelly closed her eyes and rested her head on his chest. His heart was pounding hard and fast. The festive carols ended on the CD player. They dozed off into each other's arms, dreaming of all the incredible sex games they would play on Christmas Day!

EDUARDO AND TERRI
Joseph Gaynor

She was chillin' with a couple of the guys who lived
down the street from her. They were okay. Just friends.
She'd decided to hang out that afternoon because
Manny told John, why don't they drop by to see
Eduardo at the mat on Forty-fourth? Terri knew that
Eddie had been working there for three weeks now, and
the job was almost done. This could have been one of
her last chances to really get to know him, before he had
to cut out and start working back in the city.

It was hot that day, and Manny was snapping on Terri
about how the sun was so hot, it was making her cutoff
T-shirt damp down the middle, between her sweet,
round titties.

She laughed and teased back about how skinny

Manny was, and when John slowed behind to hide from getting ranked, she grinned and let him go. John was cute, with his dark hair and B-boy good looks, but he was a little too shy for Terri's taste.

Manny called for Eduardo, who came from the darkness of the laundromat into the scorching afternoon light. Squinting, he folded his arms in front of his bare chest and offered one of those devilish killer smiles that had all the Puerto Rican girls in the 'hood just dying to meet him. Manny and John talked guy-talk, but Terri looked on and marveled at how much Eddie's body had changed.

Thick muscles had grown under the smooth tanned skin of his shoulders and upper arms. Along with the bulky muscles of his chest, they seemed to look so much bigger and stronger than she remembered. As they rapped on about John's new Mustang, Terri just tried to keep from blushing, since she was standing there and letting herself get all excited over fuckin' humpy Eduardo.

He was wearing big, heavy workman's gloves, and an old pair of paint-stained Wranglers that fit him so perfectly that it didn't matter that he'd left the front button undone and the zipper half-opened. His ass and thighs filled them to their limit and then some, she thought, taking yet another glance at the mound of his crotch. His abs had faded under a voluptuous layer of flesh.

"Hey, Eduardo, are you gettin' fat?" Terri couldn't help herself. She had to play.

246

Eddie broke off his talk with the guys and turned his ice-blue gaze at Terri. His lips broke into another of those patented wicked smiles. He leaned into the door frame in a sly, almost seductive way. Every muscle in his torso seemed to shift when he did that. His waist creased just under his heavy rib cage, pushing a meaty, sun-tanned bulge over the side of his jeans.

"Excuse me?" he said.

"Last time I saw you was at Andrea's party last April, and you were as skinny as Manny." She grinned. "You look like you put on some weight since then, so I asked you if you're getting fat, okay?"

"Why? Does it look like I'm getting fat to you, Terri?"

"I don't know...maybe you should spend less time working on washing machines and more time working out in the gym," Terri pushed a finger into Eduardo's softened but still-muscular stomach. "You're gettin' a belly!"

"Oh, shit! She dissin' my man!" Manny said.

"You gonna take that?" John laughed. Not many guys could stand up to Terri, so this was going to be good.

"What, don't you like my belly?" Eddie lowered a gloved hand to it and began rubbing. Dabs of wet paint and dirt smeared across the sweaty meat over his faded abdominals. "Don't you like my body, Terri?"

"I didn't say I didn't like your body." Terri couldn't help licking her lips. "I just said I thought you were putting on a little weight, that's all. Look at you! You can't even close your jeans."

"Yeah? Well, I think you like it that I can't close up these jeans, Terri," Eduardo's voice was deep and soft. Those ice blue eyes were boring holes into her soul. She was dripping wet. Her panties were soaked. "I think you like my jeans wide open, and I think you like guys with meat on them. Gives you something to hold on to…something to sink your teeth into. Am I right, Terri?"

"So is that why you're letting yourself get fat, Eduardo? 'Cause you know big, meaty guys, like the way you've gotten, turn me on?" Terri was getting bold, poking his torso as she spoke. "Is that where this belly came from?"

"You'll have to feed me something extra good in order to find out—won't you, Terri?"

Terri leaned into Eduardo, slipping her arms around his hot body, and leaning in to lick a bead of warm, salty sweat from his thick neck, "How about some nice pussyjuice, Eddie? I can feed you so much of that, we're gonna have to buy you a whole new pair of jeans. When I get through with you, the ones you're wearing are not gonna fit you ever again. And then, don't be surprised if you wind up being the main course on the menu, gorgeous." She slapped his fleshy sides playfully. "I might just eat you alive!"

Well, that gave Eduardo a thumping hard-on. He told the boys to meet him at the candy store down the block in fifteen minutes. He said he had something to tell Terri in private.

With the laundromat locked up from the inside, Eddie had Terri up on a washer and her tight jeans and sopping panties shucked down around her ankles in no time!

"I had to test these things out, anyway," he said, throwing a bunch of quarters into the slots and punching them in.

Before too long, the machine was humming and vibrating away, and Eddie was making good on Terri's sweet offerings. He had to laugh at how much was there. She was a cream factory, and his job was to eat everything that came out of that ripe, fruity pussy.

So he ate her, like a pig in a mountain of truffles. He licked her sloppily, slurping at her flowing juice, even as she shook and vibrated on top of the washing machine. For Terri, it was like coming forever. She squeezed his face between her thighs, and laughed and ran her hands through his close-cropped hair. She moaned in Spanish, and giggled and called him cute pet names. Reaching down over his sides, she told him she was going after his "love handles," and she grabbed and pinched that meat she'd seen bulging at his sides.

"Handle *this*, you little cocktease," Eduardo grinned.

With just two quick movements, Terri's clothes were flying, and she was off the machine and impaled on his giant cock. She was like a feather for him! All he had to do was lock her legs around his waist and simply fuck her standing straight up! Terri wrapped her arms around his powerful neck and kissed him, pausing only to let out a squeal of delight whenever he pulled her ass into him, shoving his big dick deeper inside her. She was really having a good time!

"So you wanna go out with me, Eduardo?" she asked, breathless. "We'll have a real good time. I'll make you dinner. For real—"

"I'm fucking you right here!" Eddie laughed.

"I know. Feels good!" Terri's hands slipped back down to Eddie's gut again, and he felt her nails give a warning rake under his deep-set navel. "Say yes, or I'll start tickling this pudgy belly you've gotten!"

"Yes! I'll go out with you! Jesus Christ!" he laughed. "Now it's your turn to eat! And don't spill any!"

He pulled her off his throbbing cock and dropped her gently to the floor. Without skipping a beat, she took the monster into her mouth and deep-throated him with gusto. She brought him off spectacularly, catching every spurt and relishing its salty-sweet taste. He hadn't come so much in ages, but then again, look who was making him crazy!

"C'mon, little laundry boy," she grinned, giving his sweaty, well-fed torso one last tweak. "Time to buy you some candy!"

CROSSING BOUNDARIES
Les Collins

A few months ago, my wife Susie and I had met a lovely lesbian couple who wanted to swing with a straight couple. We jumped at the opportunity. We met a couple of times, so that we could get to know one another, and decided that we were compatible. We made plans to meet at our house for our first sexual experience together.

Maggie and Alicia arrived on a Saturday evening. Being the excellent hostess that she is, my wife offered them drinks and snacks. After about an hour, everyone seemed to be completely relaxed. We made our way into the bedroom and proceeded to undress each other.

The two women jumped on the king-sized bed and bounced on it like a pair of little girls. They were very enthusiastic. Alicia parted her legs and winked at her girlfriend. Maggie crawled like a cat, wiggling her ass, toward the wet, throbbing cunt. She dove her head between her lover's legs and licked the hard moist clit, fast, then slow, then fast again. Alicia was moaning softly, her soft thighs trembling at her partner's touch.

My cock grew instantly. Susie closed her hand around my pulsating pole and stroked it gently as we watched our lesbian friends. I located my wife's protruding clit and massaged it very slowly. Her pussy was soaking wet. I felt her juices oozing out.

"Oh, baby! Suck my cunt! It feels so good! Your tongue feels so good in my pussy!" Alicia was mumbling to Maggie, having reached a state of ecstasy.

"Suck my clit into your mouth! Oh…I'm coming! I'm coming!" she exclaimed.

I couldn't believe my luck! I was standing in my bedroom, watching two gorgeous lesbians getting each other off. Susie squatted over Alicia's head. She lowered her pussy to this lovely lady's mouth. With a skilled tongue, Alicia began working my wife's cunt. I could see from Susie's expression that she was floating into the pleasure zone of no return. She was humping her cunt onto Alicia's face, pinching her own nipples as hard as she could.

All along, I was jerking my cock, waiting for the right moment to jump in. Maggie turned to me, looked at my engorged member, and slapped her firm asscheeks.

"Fuck my pussy! It's been years since a man has been there. Don't keep me waiting any longer!"

Holding my prick from the base of the shaft, I pushed

it gently into Maggie's burning snatch. Her tightness was overwhelming. She growled as I drove the swollen head into her wet opening. I held her ass and began to thrust slowly, letting her get accustomed to the feel of a red-hot, pulsating cock.

The women were lapping each other in rhythmic motions. Their movements were hypnotic. They were grunting and howling. My wife leaned forward and planted her lips on mine. We kissed over the naked bodies of the two lesbian lovers.

Alicia pulled Susie's pussylips apart and probed her hole with two fingers. Working her fingers relentlessly, in and out, brought Susie into an explosive orgasm. Her juices flowed all over Alicia's face, and she sucked them up like a hungry dog.

The three women's bodies were twisting and trembling entwined together. As much as I wanted, I couldn't hold out any longer. I thrust my strained muscle into Maggie's contracting pussy fast and hard. My balls were vibrating from the flaming come that shot through, deep into her cunt. I pumped twice more, draining my meat completely.

Gasping, I fell back on the bed, my dick still erect. Alicia, Maggie, and Susie grabbed my cock and balls and licked until I was screaming. Alicia commented on how she liked the taste of come mixed with her girlfriend's pussyjuices. Jokingly, Alicia accused Maggie of being heterosexual.

"Bite your tongue, bitch! Or, better yet, I'll bite it for you."

Maggie jumped on Alicia, and the two of them were at it again. Susie and I looked at each other, pleased that the night had just begun!

THE AUDIT
Richard Stall

The bank auditor was adding the receipts, analyzing the company's profits, and figuring out the expenses. He was intensely focused on his work.

Ms. Norris was pulling out the bookkeeping files, neatly stacking them in a pile next to him.

"It's all here for you. If there's anything else, page me."

He looked up at her as she was exiting the office. The tight rayon skirt hugged her voluptuous rump, making her crack slightly visible. His dick shifted in his pants.

"Ms. Norris, I may have a few questions for you. Please don't leave yet."

She swiveled around and strutted toward him. It seemed as if the buttons of her shirt could pop from the pressure of holding in her large, round breasts. Her nipples were protruding, pushing against the silky fabric.

Beads of sweat accumulated around his temples. His dick was swelling. Leaning over his mahogany desk, her cleavage practically pouring out, she promised to help him.

"It would not be ethical, Ms. Norris, to ask for the kind of help that I truly need right now."

"Try me!"

Pleasantly shocked at her response, he didn't hesitate to take advantage of the situation.

"My cock has a pounding headache. Is there anything you could do to soothe it?"

She kneeled between his legs, popped his zipper with her teeth, and pulled it down slowly. A nine-inch raging hard-on flew out, tapping her on the nose.

With the raspy part of her tongue, she licked the underside of his shaft, traveling all the way to the rim. With one swooping motion, her lips enveloped the swollen head. She sucked on the tip, extracting the liquid dew that had accumulated in his peehole.

He gripped the arms of his chair tightly and leaned back, thrusting his hips forward.

"Ms. Norris, I think it's working!"

Her tongue moved quickly, sideways, then up and down the shaft. Folding her hand tightly around it, she pushed down then up and over the head. She continued this motion, meanwhile, flicking her tongue under his ballbag, occasionally pulling the loose skin with her lips.

She unbuttoned her shirt, releasing her large, soft

breasts. Holding them tightly together, he slipped his cock between her cleavage. She played with her nipples as he tit-fucked her.

Pressing her chin on her chest, she stuck her tongue out. Each time his cockhead came through, she licked it. His tempo increased, and so did the lapping of her tongue.

His body tensed. His balls tightened. He shot streams of hot, milky come into her open mouth and down her tits.

When he was done, she closed her lips around the head. She sucked gently, finishing all the remains.

"Thank you, Ms. Norris. With my headache gone, I can concentrate on the company's chargebacks!"

DINNER DATE
Anthony Ronis

The doorbell rang a couple of times before I got to the buzzer. The voice through the speaker announced that Celia had arrived. I instructed my doorman to let her up.

After a couple of minutes, I heard a light knocking on the door. A tingling warmth swept my body when I opened it and laid eyes on my date. She looked stunning! Her tight short dress hugged her shapely body, accentuating every curve. Her golden California tan contrasted her long curly blonde hair that reached down the middle of her back.

I gave her a kiss on the cheek and welcomed her in. I poured drinks for both of us. Making ourselves comfortable on the large L-shaped sofa, all I could think about was getting my hands on that great body of hers.

I dipped fresh strawberries in the melted chocolate and touched her lips with it. She nibbled and chewed slowly, finishing the berry. But she didn't stop there. She licked my fingers and sucked them into her mouth. My cock twitched and shifted. With every lick of my fingers, my bulge grew bigger and bigger.

She smiled seductively and pulled me closer, practically on top of her. Our lips met and we kissed long and hard, our tongues dancing forcefully in each other's mouths. My hands brushed gently over her breasts. I began to feel her nipples. She moaned softly, her weight pushing harder against my body. I continued to squeeze her nipples until they were as hard as nails.

Suddenly she pulled away and peeled off her dress. A patch of neatly trimmed fur decorated her mound, which crowned her shaved pussylips. I grabbed her firm ass and pulled her to me. I buried my face into her hot, wet cunt, lapping up the sweet nectar dripping from her orifice.

"Oh, baby, bite my clit!"

She moaned as I obliged. She thrust her hips forward as I passed my tongue over her throbbing clit. I worked on her swollen nub until she began begging me to fuck her.

My cock had turned into a raging, pulsating muscle, dripping come. I stroked it as she sat back down and spread her legs for me.

Holding the shaft, I eased the head in. The rest followed, slowly, until my balls touched her flesh. The volume of her moans increased, and so did my speed. Celia was yelling out my name, asking me to fuck her harder, as I rammed her relentlessly.

Each time I was about to come, she dug her blood red nails into my back just enough to make me stop. Her antics made my head spin. The pressure in my balls was accumulating.

"I want you to come in my ass!"

Celia's request was too good to pass up. I pulled my red-hot cock out of her cunt, flipped her over, and prepared for rear entry. Bent over doggy-style, she reached back to spread her asscheeks so that I could see her little puckered hole better. Her thoughtfulness touched me.

I rested my cockhead in her crack and pushed slowly. Since my dick had been well lubricated by her pussyjuices, mixed with my precome fluid, it slipped in painlessly. Her hole was tight and burning hot. I held firmly onto her hips and pumped her ass, slow at first then a bit faster.

My thick, large cock pushing into her tight, narrow passage, created an intense friction. Celia was fingering her cunt and rubbing her pussy, grunting and growling as I thrust into her. My pulsating prick was becoming increasingly sensitive.

She continued working on her clit and pussyhole until she came—screaming to God, her body convulsing—then screaming to me, her pussy contracting!

I gave her ass ten more strokes. My balls tensed and bunched up, trying to push a load of hot steamy come through, finally exploding with great force, sending a jet of creamy liquid, deep into her stretched rectum.

As I pulled out my meat, droplets of my milky come

oozed out of her sphincter. I massaged it around her hole, pushing some of it back in with my finger.

Her body went limp and she leaned forward, resting on the sofa's back. As I collapsed next to her, trying to catch my breath, I realized that dinner was getting cold.

I had the whole evening planned. First we had to have dinner. Then we were gonna have dessert. Afterward, I was gonna prime her all over again for the second round of fucking. I wasn't letting her leave the apartment until every orifice had been thoroughly screwed. And as far as I could see, there were at least two more to go!

MILKY MAIDEN
Anais Contreau

Thinking that she was alone, Melinda stood in front of the living room wall mirror, unbuttoning her peach satin dress. The flames of the two lit candles flickered, highlighting the copper tones of her thick, long, curly hair. When the last button was undone, she let the dress fall to the floor, leaving her body bare except for her high-heeled shoes.

She wore a gold ankle bracelet with a tiny bell that chimed when she moved. Her legs were long and sleek, silky to the touch. Her creamy thighs and firm rounded bottom looked absolutely delicious. Her prominent pubic mound was decorated with tight little curls that ended right at the crease where her fleshy pussylips united. Her rounded hips curved smoothly into her small, dainty waist.

Gently brushing her long red fingernails over her flat tummy, up her sides, tracing her barely noticeable ribs, she stopped under the curves of her large, round breasts. They were firm and sloped upward, garnished with a set of thick dark pink nipples.

Watching her reflection in the golden light, she weighed her breasts in her hands and was satisfied with how heavy they felt. Moving to a tray nearby, she greased her hands with a rose-scented body oil and spread the warm liquid across her tits. Massaging each of them gently, she thrilled to the feel of herself, and the way her hard nipples felt under her palms.

If she played with her nipples long and hard enough, sometimes small droplets of milk would ooze out of them. Just doing that could bring her close to orgasm.

As she continued to squeeze her now-swollen nipples, she noticed a shadowy reflection in the mirror. She tried to focus her eyes on the image, but it was too late. Two large masculine hands surrounded her waist and traveled up her body. They enveloped her breasts, palms sliding roughly against her stiffened nipples. Melinda gasped and tried to get away.

"Relax," his deep voice whispered in her ear. "I'm not going to hurt you. I've been watching you for some time now. I know what you like."

Melinda shivered, goose bumps spreading across the tender flesh of her body like a cold fire. But, like a fever dream, the stroking of his warm hands somehow soothed her. She leaned back against his naked torso and relaxed, allowing herself to be embraced by his muscular arms.

Images of a dozen men flashed through her mind: an ex-boyfriend, the handsome stud next door, the mailman who'd caught her in her negligee the other morning. She could see in the mirror that he was a large man, but his face was still hidden in the shadows.

The mystery of his identity mixed with her fear and added a new dimension to her excitement. She leaned into him as he began to fondle and squeeze her breasts gently. His fingers swirled around her rockhard nipples.

She moaned softly, pressing the back of her head against his chest. He pushed her hair to the side and nibbled on her ear, pulling on it with his tongue, drawing it delicately into his mouth. He pushed his hips forward, positioning his massive hard-on at the crack of her ass. Her apprehension kept her all but frozen, but she desired more.

With one hand, he parted her pussylips and stroked her moist, throbbing clit a couple of times before he began toying with her burning, wet hole. She bit her lips in a failed effort to restrain her whimpering.

"I know you like this," he murmured. "If you don't, tell me to stop, and I will."

Melinda kept quiet, and his fingers continued to push in and out of her velvety pussy. He lubricated her nipples with her juice, and even drew a trail of it from her lips to her navel. He seemed to know all of her sweet spots: her aureoles, the small of her back, the curve of her belly just above her mons Veneris. Already, a powerful orgasm was building deep between her thighs, ready to wash over her, spurred by the adrenaline rush of being alone in her living room with a strange and powerful man.

His handiwork paid off. Small droplets of milky nectar had begun to form on her nipples. And when he realized what was happening, he moved to draw more of it. He continued squeezing, keeping her nipples stiff, until more of the translucent white fluid appeared. He turned her around, and, taking the full weight of her breasts in his hands, he pushed them into his mouth and suckled until her moans turned into growls.

"Get on your knees!"

She listened to him without uttering a word. Now she was facing his raging hard-on. It must've been a good nine or ten inches long, thick as a jungle snake. The head was fat, with a pronounced rim, and a tiny pool of precome glistened in his peehole.

"Make it good and wet!" His whisper had grown hoarse with lust.

Circling the rim with her tongue, she sipped his fluid and closed her lips tight around the head. She drew it in very slowly.

"Put your hands behind your back!"

She followed his instructions, never stopping to ask questions. He held her head in position and pumped in a slow rhythm, her mouth being forced to open wider to accommodate his engorged prick. She almost couldn't help allowing her teeth to scrape the taut skin of his shaft.

Perfectly still, now, taking him in, she gazed up at him, trying to focus on his shadowy face. She could see nothing.

The grip around her head tightened and his tempo increased. His back arched, and he began to grunt like an animal. Finally, pulling forcefully out of her mouth, he stroked his cock roughly five or six more times—and detonated his load, shooting streams and streams of thick hot come all over her large, sweaty breasts.

He gasped for air and tried to catch his breath. A few seconds of silence passed.

"Get up!"

His whisper was as firm as ever. She stood in front of him her eyes trailing the beads of sweat trailing down his torso. He rubbed his hot come all around her tits, completely coating her sore nipples. He pushed her tits together and then up to her mouth.

"Now suck my milk."

Fixing her eyes into the shadows beneath his brow, she took both nipples into her mouth and sucked them, swallowing his bitter come mixed with the delectable sweetness of her milk.

He pulled her tits out of her mouth and kissed her lips, licking the white film around them.

"I'll be back when it's time to feed you again."

He stepped back into the shadows and disappeared without a trace.

NUMBER 6 UPTOWN
Julian Anthony Guerra

By Lex everyone had left the car but me and the couple
—who'd wanna stay in there when it was so amazingly
hot? Me, I stayed, readin' the paper, but not carefully,
'cause my gaze kept drifting to that girl. She had such
nice red lips, her butt seemed planted firmly in her
boyfriend's hand, all pulled up close to him. He was
Latino (her too, probably), and he relaxed and closed his
eyes. A red belt cinched the billowy white blouse she
wore, the hem was pushed up in back where his fingers
lay into the curve of her ass. A few moments before,
she'd placed her hand casually on his left upper thigh,
and it was still there, just under his waist, near his
crotch.

His shirt open down his chest, his St. Christopher

269

medal glinting over his broad pecs, he didn't mind where her hand was at, what-so-ever. He was muscular, his arms filling out his short sleeves till they tightened around his biceps. He'd managed to push himself into a pair of gray-black two-tones that encased his thick thighs and squeezed at his torso. Stiflin' a smirk, I noticed the denim'd pulled a bit over his mound—she'd been tickling at him in a lazy, sleepy way with her fingertips for minutes now, and every once in a while, she'd lean over and kiss his face or nuzzle his neck or somethin', turning him on (definitely!) with those sweet red lips and that moist tongue that slipped out between them.

Before too long, she must have forgotten I was there (or didn't care), but slowly she started to rub her hand over his cockbulge, making it bigger while she sucked and bit his neck. With his smooth features and thick eyebrows, he barely seemed to notice! (At least that's how he was making it look!)

He must have liked it, though. His hand tightened around the softness of her rump, exciting her, making her blush. Next, she put both hands to work, and she had this little smile on as they slid down the front of his belly. Now she was scrunching up the cotton and spreading away the sides from out of his jeans. She hugged him, slipping an arm around his solid back so that her nails dug into the beef at his side before clasping with her other hand. Kissing him again, she touched his navel and the swell of dark skin that pinched over his two-tones.

She whispered somethin' in his ear and a brow went

up. She giggled, tap-kissing his chest and prodding the meat of his belly playfully. He laughed, arching his body like a big jungle cat. Then she popped the button of his jeans open.

His dick was long and hard, she went down on it right away. She got it all into her mouth, and down her wet throat all at once. Nodding up and down, she sucked him as they held each other, leaving slick saliva to dribble down his shaft into his pants.

Pulling the zipper all the way down, tugging at him, licking his big meat, she made him gasp and moan in Spanish, his hips rotatin' back-'n'-forth. She blew him like I'd never seen. It was a blowjob supreme. Fit for a king.

The load he finally shot was so big and creamy, her cheeks filled before she could swallow every drop. Some of that white-hot come oozed from her lips, and she had to use his shirttail to wipe her smiling face clean.

Don't know whether the group of hungry-eyed *chicanas* who got on the next stop could get enough of him, or the big ol' straight-iron in my pants!

THE BUTCHER SHOP
Olga Mathersby

"Hey, Louie—look who just walked in! It's Gina the bombshell!"

"Wipe down the counter, Manny, and button your lip."

"Sure thing, boss."

"I want your most tender piece of veal—and make sure it's fresh!"

"Only the best for my number-one customer! If it's not fresh, it's not from Louie's!"

"I don't see any veal in the freezer. Are you hiding it?"

"I just got a delivery this morning. Come around the back and you can pick out the best piece of meat I've got. Manny, take over with the customers."

"Gina, follow me!"

"Where're we goin'?"

"Back here—I got the best meat, saved up just for you! Lean beef, tender veal. It just came in."

"Don't look so fresh to me!"

"Ah, c'mon, Gina, don't say that about my meat!"

"I'm tellin' ya, I've seen better!"

"Yeah? Where?"

"Well, for instance, Louie, right there, between those legs."

"Gina, you're…embarrassing me!"

"Yeah, right! I don't think anything could embarrass you. Look at that big, fat hard-on you got."

"Well what guy could help himself with you in the room? You're a knockout!"

"Let me take a look at that juicy piece of beefsteak."

"Here! Sink your teeth into that!"

"Mmmmm, that looks real good. I never expected it to be so thick! It must be over nine inches long. I'd love to stuff myself with that."

"This'll satisfy any starved woman. Once you chow down on my cock, you'll be totally satisfied."

"Come here, Louie. Lemme lick the tip of your cockhead. I want to feel the rim of it under my tongue. I want to taste your salty precome!"

"Let me see your tongue. Here you go. Take it in your mouth. Close your lips around that dick. Yeah… like that. Lick it all 'round with your tongue…that's it."

"Mmmm, it feels so good in my mouth. It's so warm on my tongue. I just wanna gobble it up! Mmm…"

"Faster! Suck on it harder—oh, yeah! That feels great!"

"Stand up, Gina. Let me take off that blouse."

"Go ahead. I'll help you."

"Oh, your tits are so full...round. Look at those hot nipples. Delicious! Tender little vittles. Let's see how hard they can get. Is that squeezing too hard?"

"No, it feels great. Rub them between your thumbs and forefingers. Pull them gently."

"I'd like to taste you, too. I'm gonna nibble on these sweeties!"

"Yeah, Louie, that feels great! Flick your tongue on 'em. Lick 'em up real fast!"

"Anything for my best customer. You're gettin' a wet pussy there—did you know that? Matter of fact, it's soaked. Look at this juice on my fingers. Mmmm...tasty!"

"I think my pussy's ready for something much bigger than your fingers. I'd like to feel that big, pulsing muscle ram its way up there!"

"Put your leg up on this stool and spread as far out as you can. That's it! Tilt your cunt toward me. There you go! You're such a good girl!"

"Louie, I'm not gonna be able to keep my balance."

"Don't worry about it! Come to Papa. I'll carry you. Stand on your tippy-toes. There, Gina. Let me squeeze those firm asscheeks of yours."

"That feels good! Pull my cheeks apart and touch me there."

"That's quite a tight little asshole you got there. Maybe I could loosen it up with my finger... It's a persistent little hole, just wants to stay shut. I'll just have to push a little harder!"

"Oh, God, that feels great! Push it deeper! I want to feel it all around, inside my asshole."

"Wait a minute! My cock is lonely. It's so hard, it hurts! I need to give it a little company...and some tight friction action. Here's the head for a start."

"*Oh!* Please Louie, stick it in! All the way! God I wannit all the way in!"

"Well, then, here! Take the rest of it. Oh, yeah... you're so fuckin' tight. I love it! Your pussy's so hot and wet!"

"Keep sucking on my nipples, Louie! You can bite down a little harder. Pull them with your teeth. I think...I'm...gonna come!"

"Yeah baby, come for Papa! Let me feel those juices on my cock...let me feel your burning-hot pussy coming on my dick!"

"Don't stop, Louie...keep that prick of yours pumping! I wanna feel my pussy get sore!"

"Take it hard then, Gina! Can you handle that? Or should I just keep fucking you harder and harder?"

"Fuck harder and harder! I want my pussy raw!"

"I'm gonna come!"

"Come, baby...spill it for me!"

"I'm gonna explode all over you! I'm gonna squirt deep in your cunt, and then all over those big round tits of yours!"

"Give it to me...I wannit in my mouth...I wanna taste your thick creamy come!"

"Aaaaaahhh!"

"Yes, Louie! Come into me! Come!"

"Oh, man! There…take it in your mouth, Gina. Swallow it! Man! My balls are killing me! …There, on your tits…wipe it on your pussy…rub it on your throbbing clit!"

"It's all over me, Louie. It's even between my fingers! Mmmm…I'm gonna swallow every bit of it!"

"Oh, man, Gina! I love that!"

"I must say, Louie, you *do* have the best, freshest piece of meat!"

"What did I tell you? If it ain't from Louie's, it ain't fresh! And I always give the very best to my number one customer!"

BROOKSIDE
Sean Masters

He stands there, brown in the sun, teeth dazzling, his white shirt open, untucked, hands in pockets, curly brown hair dripping, leaning against a tree.

She struggles, balancing, slipping a wet calf into dry denim, nude above her waist. Inches of beaded, gleaming thigh stand firm in protest to the slowly rising fabric. Buttocks cheeks quiver uneasily as they are lowered, then pressed into their slings. Swiveling her hips, she draws a breath through glossy lips, tries to fill her lungs.

His grin broadens, his fingers absently skimming his own torso as her breasts rise. The bone and muscle of her body has been adorned with a rich and creamy flesh. Curving with a fullness that was at once lean and sumptuous, she was irresistible.

Arms and golden shoulders working, buttons are pulled closed one at a time. A moment passes, and the delicate swell of her cool belly has been scooped and smoothened.

Mercifully, a snap is left undone, and a buttery naveled waist is left free to simmer in the afternoon heat.

He moves to kiss her, and she receives him. Before long they are both back in the brook, from whence they came.

They embrace against the chill of the water. He feels her body wet against his, and it makes him large with passion. She pulls his shirt around them, but it does precious little to veil their impending union.

She kisses his chest, and he caresses her face. She allows him into her, and he fills her so, that it feels as if she were indulging in an enormous and most satisfying meal.

Plump and flush in his arms, he holds her close and moves into her repeatedly, thrusting to the strains of rushing waters and windblown leaves.

They draw of one another's breath, taste of one another's mouths. The nubs of their teats strike sparks of pleasure as they move to tighten their union.

Their call rises to join the cries of birds in the birches, the wind over the highest tops of surrounding conifers.

Treading to shore, they move slowly toward yet another mournfully doomed attempt at donning their clothes and making for civilization.

ROCK JERSEY
Robert Janelli

The gorgeous black-haired girl with luscious thick-nippled tits and a pouting round ass pulled the shirttail of her faded Metallica jersey from the low sling of her tight-fitting blue jeans. Its thready lower edge now lay over her crotch, moist from where it had been bunched between her thighs by cream that had been seeping from within her panties since he had stepped up to her.

She was so turned on by the way he looked that she had popped a small orgasm just by pulling her shirt from the torn and faded denim. Her pussylips were actually swollen to the bursting point with excitement and were so hungry for some nice cock that they actually seemed to pull her hips toward him. It felt as if her sweet snatch was about to tear through its silk and denim package just to get hold of him, pull open his dungarees, and begin sucking down his meat. There would be plenty to savor, gulp, gobble and swallow, but she would take her time, teasing him along, making him work for it.

Sliding a hand up from her leg, he brushed gently over the pussy dampness on the edge of her rock jersey, then slowly hiked the soft cotton fabric up over her waist.

To look at the bottom quarter moons of her juicy, trembling breasts, that fleshy tender torso, that sweet navel planted so deeply over the gentle swell of her golden belly; to look at all of this caused his body to tense, his breath to grow shallow with desire.

He found himself kissing her mouth, slipping his tongue into its soft wetness. Plucking her jeans open, he folded them down around her thighs, peeling her slowly, easily, like a long, plump, sun-ripened grape. Fingering her soaking pussy, he listened as her own breath grew irregular, frantic.

His lips firmly working at hers, he suddenly felt her hands wringing his waist, their fingernails catching wildly on the fabric of his T-shirt, ripping it down from around his body, violently furrowing the warm muscular skin beneath. Tugging at him, she exposed a cock, purple and swollen to the bursting point. There—where they stood—she pushed it up into her crotch.

The plunge was hot and syrupy, soft and tight. He was still kissing her, even as her nails continued raking his T-shirt to ribbons. He pumped her, fucking her up against a wall, sinking it hard enough to hear that pouty ass of hers slap rhythmically against the plaster. Moaning loudly with pleasure, he finally came, firing jets of hot semen into her steaming vagina. Sliding him down to her broiling pussy, she made him gorge on the leftovers.

QUARTERBACK'S LUCK
Teddy Lazarus

Darryl was sitting at the bus stop reading his sports magazine, sipping his grape soda. The sun was beating down on him, and the bus was taking forever. Even the article about his favorite football star couldn't calm his impatience. His annoyance with the public-transportation system was building up.

A loud honking broke his concentration. He looked up, only to see Katie in her cherry red convertible.

"Hey, Darryl, what're you doing?"

"Yo, Katie wassup? I'm just waitin' for the bus."

"You need a ride?"

Darryl was shocked. A hot blonde blue-eyed college cheerleader had just offered a big black guy a ride!

"Hop on in, Darryl! What are you waiting for?"

He looked her in the eye and, with slight apprehension, he walked over leisurely and got in her car.

"Where to Mr. Quarterback?"

"I'm just going to practice, but I'll be two hours early by car. I had it timed for the bus."

"Then let's go to my dorm for some cold beers!"

"Wow, that sounds great! I guess Coach won't mind if I have only one."

Katie was focused on the road ahead, and Darryl was focused on Katie's large, round softball tits. They would jiggle just the right way when she jumped up and down, cheering at the games. Her long legs and firm ass had always given all the guys something to talk about. He was drooling mentally about the things he wanted to do to her.

"Okay, we're here."

His lusty fantasy shattered at the sound of her words. Darryl followed Katie into the dorm and up to her room. There was a bed, a chair, and a little ice-box inside. He chose the chair, and Katie handed him a bottle of beer.

She sat on the bed and sipped straight from the bottle. Darryl kept his gaze on her, even as he chugalugged his beer. Her long, silky blonde hair, smooth creamy skin, big firm tits, was more than enough to make his cock swell.

"So why you bein' so nice to me? What you want? 'Cause a girl like you don't just invite a guy like me to her place without wanting somethin'!"

"I think you're a nice guy, and I like you."

"You like me!?"

"Yeah, is that so hard to believe?"

"Sugar, you don't *know* me well enough to like me! Maybe it's something else you want. Maybe it's my big black dick!"

"Uh...Darryl..."

"Don't 'uh Darryl' me! You drive me to your place, give me a beer, tell me that you like me.... You want my dick, bitch—and I'm gonna give it to you!"

Before she had a chance to say a word, he was standing in front of her, giant ebony hard-on in his hand, stroking it an inch away from her face.

The length and thickness of Darryl's enormous cock left her speechless. She was almost hypnotized by it. He tapped her luscious lips with the tip. She gave a slight startled jump and looked up at him.

"What're you waitin' for? Take it in your mouth, baby...."

Her gaze switched back down to his monstrous erection. Parting her lips slightly, a reluctant tongue peered out, swiping a quick lick at the drooling precome. She opened wider, and Darryl pushed the head into her salivating mouth. Katie's lips sealed around the rim, and her tongue circled the area just around the peehole. She sucked the head a couple of times and then took the shaft.

Darryl's cock was so immense that her mouth was full, and it was only halfway in! Holding his cock steady with her delicate hands, she licked and nibbled up and down the sides.

Darryl was holding her by her hair, pushing her head

forward gently. She worked her way down to his balls and licked the sac in the middle, trailing her tongue right under. Darryl's head tilted back, his eyes closed, and hips thrust slightly forward. He licked his lips in anticipation of things to come.

Katie sucked one ball into her mouth, then the other. She rolled them gently around and poured them out again. She was getting hornier by the second. Darryl pulled his jersey off, exposing his thick, muscular arms and chest. His skin was smooth and shiny, with a few curly hairs in the middle of his chest.

Katie admired his strong well-built physique. He reached down to her and pushed her shoulders back. She responded to his gesture by leaning back on the bed.

Taking his time, he unbuttoned her shirt. She was braless. Her large tits had a ruddy glow, and her pinkish nipples were puckered hard. He cupped her breasts and squeezed them, making the nipples protrude even more. He fondled one, while sucking and tugging on the other.

Spreading her fleshy white thighs, Darryl mounted her and rubbed his hard cock on her furry mound. Katie tightened her ass muscles and tilted her hips up. His cock slid down between her pussylips. He rubbed it on her moist, throbbing clit. Their breathing was fast and heavy, almost synchronized.

He located her wet tight opening with his cockhead, positioned and pushed in very slowly. The entrance took her breath away. She gasped and dug her nails into his back, his dick stretching her small hole to new limits.

Once he was in all the way, he held still. Darryl

lowered his head and kissed her. Their tongues wrestled wildly, and he began pumping her tight hot pussy. He grunted with every deep thrust, chewing her lips, her neck, her tits.

Katie was moaning and growling, her body trembling and shuddering under his weight. He cupped her meaty asscheeks with his large rough hands and up pushed her hips. His speed increased. She screamed out his name over and over, as her pussy contracted around his pulsating cock. He thrust harder, giving her orgasm after orgasm.

Katie wrapped her lips around his massive thighs and squeezed her pussy muscles, giving him maximum friction. Pushing her huge tits into his mouth, Darryl suckled on them as he fucked her forcefully.

Darryl's body tensed, his balls tightened, and his cock exploded violently. Katie's cunt was flooded with loads of thick milky come. He continued pumping into her sloppy pussy, the fluids oozing out of her hole, and down the crack of her ass.

He pulled his cock out of her cunt and rubbed it on her tummy. He rolled over and landed on his back next to her. Katie grasped onto his semierect dick and licked off his sticky come, mixed with her pussyjuices. She wiped all around his shaft and balls with her tongue, cleaning up every drop.

"Ah, baby…that was good, but I gotta get ready for training."

"Are you gonna have energy?"

"No, but I'll just think of my cheerleader's pink pussy, and that'll give me the stamina to go on!"

THICKER THAN WATER
Amelio Tancero

Since our last meeting, my second cousin Rachel had developed into a stunning young woman. She had a curvaceous bod, high, rounded breasts, long legs, and a killer smile.

When she was just a kid, I'd tease her viciously. She followed me around everywhere, only to be humiliated or, even worse, ignored. Now the tables had turned. I wanted to follow *her* around everywhere! I was lucky, though. Her sweet nature hadn't changed, and she was eager to spend her free time with me and get reacquainted.

I invited Rachel over to see my first apartment since I'd moved from my parents' home. It was my very own bachelor pad, and man, I felt like a king! Rachel arrived promptly at eight that night with a bottle of champagne. I couldn't get over the fact that my younger cousin was now old enough to buy liquor!

I showed her around the studio, which took a long five minutes, and we sat on my cheesy sofa-bed, reminiscing about old times. Trying to be suave, I popped the champagne cork, and sparkling wine spilled all over us, soaking our clothes. Luckily, there was plenty left to drink.

I gave her a terry-cloth robe, and I changed into a pair of shorts. We talked and drank until we were slightly tipsy. Rachel even stopped trying to keep the loose robe from opening around her chest. Trying hard not to notice, I kept trying to avert my eyes, but my cock shifted in my shorts. I tried to stay loose and casual, but I failed as usual, and she started noticing that something was up!

I had to confess.

"Rachel, I know you're my cousin and all, but I think you've grown into quite a babe! I haven't felt this strongly about any other woman."

"Jack, I'm flattered! I think you're kind of a hunk yourself. But then again, I always felt that way about you!"

Lady luck was smiling down on me. I touched her face gently. Her skin was silky soft. I leaned over and gave her a light kiss on her luscious full lips. Rachel responded by kissing me back. Our tongues met and we explored each other's mouths enthusiastically. Her sweet scent and taste were maddening to me.

I slipped my hand under the robe and caressed her breasts. Rachel moaned softly and pressed her body against mine. I had a raging hard-on.

"Rachel, you're making me so hot it hurts."

"Let me make it better for you."

My cock almost exploded when her warm, soft hand folded around my throbbing shaft. With a feathery touch, she stroked my cock, rolling her palm over my dripping cockhead. I eased her back on the bed and continued to kiss her as she played with my dick.

I removed my robe and with I suckled on her hard pink nipples. Rachel gasped. I felt her body tremble at my touch. I put my hand on her tummy and rubbed my way down to her mound. I tugged gently on her neatly trimmed fur and parted her juicy pussylips. I teased her clitoris, tapping on the little peak with the tip of my finger, feeling it swell.

Rachel moaned and parted her legs slightly. I mounted her and brushed the head of my cock up and down her clit. Her opening was soaking wet.

"Come on, Jack, don't make your little cousin wait. Stick it in my pussy and make me come!"

"Anything for you, babe."

I pushed the head in and, as she growled, I pushed the shaft all the way. I shoved it in until my balls pressed against her asscheeks. Her cunt was hot and tight. I pumped slowly at first. Then I fucked her faster and harder. It didn't matter that she was my second cousin. I didn't care who anyone was anymore. I was delirious with ecstasy.

"Fuck me harder, baby. C'mon, Jack—fuck me harder!"

"I'll fuck you raw. I'll pump that pussy till you scream!"

Rachel was kneading my torso and sides, pushing her body up to meet my thrusts. She was screaming out my name, telling me how good I made her feel, when her body tensed and began to spasm.

Her twitching and trembling made me crazy. Her pussy muscles were convulsing around my dick, increasing the friction. My balls felt like they were gonna burst. I gave her a couple more strokes—and shot a heavy load deep into her pussy. I continued to pump until I had nothing—and I mean *nothing*—left to give. I pulled it out and rested beside her.

Rachel gave me a kiss and thanked me for showing her my bachelor pad…and my cock. We hugged and kissed and finished the bottle of champagne. My apartment was thoroughly broken in, and so was my cousin!

STRANGE PICKUP

Julian Anthony Guerra

At a neighborhood bar, a guy pulls up to me and orders a beer. He turns to ask me the time and I tell him it's early. He grins pleasantly and drinks up. I notice he's good-looking and fairly well built. In fact, the fit of his T-shirt reveals both thick, sinewy arm and shoulder muscles, as well as a gentle hint of softness low around his waist, like he was an ex-jock just settling in to married life.

We get to talking. He looks—shyly at times—into my eyes and touches my arm, and I take to him quickly. He shows me a picture of his girlfriend, a gorgeous country-girl brunette in a tube top and miniskirt, and invites me home to meet her. I allow myself to go for this and believe his sincerity.

In the kitchen of their house, I can't help but to ogle her as she fixes us sandwiches. In shorts and a western-style halter, she looks twice as good as she did in the picture. She had clearly expected her guy to bring home someone, since she treated me like gold and began slowly to mess with him in ways that were sure to turn on anyone.

The way he moved her as she bent over to kiss him showed me every luscious curve, from her thighs to her ass, to her flat belly and big round breasts. They looked so good there in front of me with their tongues in each other's mouths and fingers in each other's shirts. Frankly, I wouldn't have minded joining in.

I realized I was going to get my hands on that girl about thirty seconds after he showed me her picture in the bar. Now I see how he's going to have me do it. I guess I don't mind.

She leads me onto their bed, where I kneel to face her. The nipples on her luscious breasts have hardened and are almost touching me through the fabric of her halter. His breath is warm and easy on my neck, and I feel his hands move firmly around to the front of my torso to unbutton my jeans and lift my T-shirt.

She unzips me, spreads apart the denim, and pulls out my raging hard-on, licking my chest and stomach as she does. I feel a little funny about her boyfriend holding me so tightly while she goes to work on me, but then I figure it's too late now, so I decide to relax and enjoy it.

Pretty soon he's delivering powerful kisses over the nape of my neck and my shoulders! I would have tried to stop him, or say something at least, but the blowjob she'd started giving me was so stunning that I couldn't even move. She's kneading my asscheeks, sliding the nails of her thumbs up the softness of my underbelly, as my shaft is repeatedly gulped and suckled to the root.

The feel of her silky hair bobbing against me, her wriggling tongue sliding up and down my pulsing meat, his body wrapped around me from behind, the sound of all that quiet slurping—it all made me rise up into a spasm, and made my come go flying. I shot my load into her face and watched it flow down her neck and onto her breasts, even as I continued to come. The weirdness, the fantastic blowjob, that silky blonde hair dancing against me, I just kept shooting and coming.

They gave me their number after it was over and asked me to call them sometime. It's been a while, and I haven't had the courage. I think about it a lot, though.

MASQUERADE BOOKS

MASQUERADE

VISCOUNT LADYWOOD
GYNECOCRACY
$7.95/511-5
Julian, whose parents feel he shows just a bit too much spunk, is sent to a very special private school, in hopes that he will learn to discipline his wayward soul. Once there, Julian discovers that his program of study has been devised by the deliciously stern Mademoiselle de Chambonnard. In no time, Julian is learning the many ways of pleasure—under the firm hand of this demanding headmistress.

EDITED BY CHARLOTTE ROSE
50 PLAYGIRL FANTASIES
$6.50/460-7
A steamy selection of women's fantasies straight from the pages of *Playgirl*—the leading magazine of sexy entertainment for women. These tales of seduction—specially selected by no less an authority than Charlotte Rose, author of such bestselling women's erotica as *Women at Work* and *The Doctor is In*—are sure to set your pulse racing.

N. T. MORLEY
THE PARLOR
$6.50/496-8
Lovely Kathryn gives in to the ultimate temptation. The mysterious John and Sarah ask her to be their slave—an idea that turns Kathryn on so much that she can't refuse! But who are these two mysterious strangers? Little by little, Kathryn not only learns to serve, but comes to know the inner secrets of her stunning keepers.

JULIAN ANTHONY GUERRA, EDITOR
COME QUICKLY:
FOR COUPLES ON THE GO
$6.50/461-5
The increasing pace of daily life is no reason to forgo a little carnal pleasure whenever the mood strikes. Here are over sixty of the hottest fantasies around—all designed to get you going in less time than it takes to dial 976. A superhot volume especially for couples on a modern schedule.

ERICA BRONTE
LUST, INC.
$6.50/467-4
Lust, Inc. explores the extremes of passion that lurk beneath even the coldest, most business-like exteriors. Join in the sexy escapades of a group of high-powered professionals whose idea of office decorum is like nothing you've ever encountered! Business attire not required....

VANESSA DURIES
THE TIES THAT BIND
$6.50/510-7
The incredible confessions of a thrillingly unconventional woman. From the first page, this chronicle of dominance and submission will keep you gasping with its vivid depictions of sensual abandon. At the hand of Masters Georges, Patrick, Pierre and others, this submissive seductress experiences pleasures she never knew existed....

M. S. VALENTINE
THE CAPTIVITY OF CELIA
$6.50/453-6
Colin is mistakenly considered the prime suspect in a murder, forcing him to seek refuge with his cousin, Sir Jason Hardwicke. In exchange for Colin's safety, Jason demands Celia's unquestioning submission—knowing she will do anything to protect her lover. Sexual extortion!

AMANDA WARE
BOUND TO THE PAST
$6.50/452-6
Anne accepts a research assignment in a Tudor mansion. Upon arriving, she finds herself aroused by James, a descendant of the mansion's owners. Together they uncover the perverse desires of the mansion's long-dead master—desires that bind Anne inexorably to the past—not to mention the bedpost!

SACHI MIZUNO
SHINJUKU NIGHTS
$6.50/493-3
Another tour through the lives and libidos of the seductive East, from the author of *Passion in Tokyo*. No one is better that Sachi Mizuno at weaving an intricate web of sensual desire, wherein many characters are ensnared and enraptured by the demands of their long-denied carnal natures. One by one, each surrenders social convention for the unashamed pleasures of the flesh.
PASSION IN TOKYO
$6.50/454-2
Tokyo—one of Asia's most historic and seductive cities. Come behind the closed doors of its citizens, and witness the many pleasures that await. Lusty men and women from every stratum of Japanese society free themselves of all inhibitions. ...

MARTINE GLOWINSKI
POINT OF VIEW
$6.50/433-X
With the assistance of her new, unexpectedly kinky lover, she discovers and explores her exhibitionist tendencies—until there is virtually nothing she won't do before the horny audiences her man arranges! Unabashed acting out for the sophisticated voyeur.

MASQUERADE BOOKS

RICHARD McGOWAN
A HARLOT OF VENUS
$6.50/425-9

A highly fanciful, epic tale of lust on Mars! Cavortia—the most famous and sought-after courtesan in the cosmopolitan city of Venus—finds love and much more during her adventures with some of the most remarkable characters in recent erotic fiction.

M. ORLANDO
THE ARCHITECTURE OF DESIRE
Introduction by Richard Manton
$6.50/490-9

Two novels in one special volume! In *The Hotel Justine*, an elite clientele is afforded the opportunity to have any and all desires satisfied. *The Villa Sin* is inherited by a beautiful woman who soon realizes that the legacy of the ancestral estate includes bizarre erotic ceremonies. Two pieces of prime real estate.

CHET ROTHWELL
KISS ME, KATHERINE
$5.95/410-0

Beautiful Katherine can hardly believe her luck. Not only is she married to the charming and oh-so-agreeable Nelson, she's free to live out all her erotic fantasies with other men. Katherine has discovered Nelson to be far more devoted than the average spouse—and the duo soon begin exploring a relationship more demanding than marriage!

MARCO VASSI
THE STONED APOCALYPSE
$5.95/401-1/mass market

"Marco Vassi is our champion sexual energist." —VLS
During his lifetime, Marco Vassi praised by writers as diverse as Gore Vidal and Norman Mailer, and his reputation was worldwide. *The Stoned Apocalypse* is Vassi's autobiography; chronicling a cross-country trip on America's erotic byways, it offers a rare glimpse of a generation's sexual imagination.

ROBIN WILDE
TABITHA'S TEASE
$5.95/387-2

When poor Robin arrives at The Valentine Academy, he finds himself subject to the torturous teasing of Tabitha—the Academy's most notoriously domineering co-ed. But Tabitha is pledge-mistress of a secret sorority dedicated to enslaving young men. Robin finds himself the utterly helpless (and wildly excited) captive of Tabitha & Company's weird desires! A marathon of ticklish torture!

ERICA BRONTE
PIRATE'S SLAVE
$5.95/376-7

Lovely young Erica is stranded in a country where lust knows no bounds. Desperate to escape, she finds herself trading her firm, luscious body to any and all men willing and able to help her. Her adventure has its ups and downs, ins and outs—all to the undeniable pleasure of lusty Erica!

CHARLES G. WOOD
HELLFIRE
$5.95/358-9

A vicious murderer is running amok in New York's sexual underground—and Nick O'Shay, a virile detective with the NYPD, plunges deep into the case. He soon becomes embroiled in an elusive world of fleshly extremes, hunting a madman seeking to purge America with fire and blood sacrifices. Set in New York's infamous sexual underground.

OLIVIA M. RAVENSWORTH
THE MISTRESS OF CASTLE ROHMENSTADT
$5.95/372-4

Lovely Katherine inherits a secluded European castle from a mysterious relative. Upon arrival she discovers, much to her delight, that the castle is a haven of sensual pleasure. Katherine learns to shed her inhibitions and enjoy her new home's many delights. Soon, Castle Rohmenstadt is the home of every perversion known to man.

CLAIRE BAEDER, EDITOR
LA DOMME: A DOMINATRIX ANTHOLOGY
$5.95/366-X

A steamy smorgasbord of female domination! Erotic literature has long been filled with heartstopping portraits of domineering women, and now the most memorable have been brought together in one beautifully brutal volume. A must for all fans of true Woman Power.

TINY ALICE
THE GEEK
$5.95/341-4

"An accomplishment of which anybody may be proud." —Philip José Farmer
The Geek is told from the point of view of a chicken, who reports on the various perversities he witnesses as part of a traveling carnival. When a gang of renegade lesbians kidnaps Chicken and his geek, all hell breaks loose.

CHARISSE VAN DER LYN
SEX ON THE NET
$5.95/399-6

Electrifying erotica from one of the Internet's hottest and most widely read authors. Encounters of all kinds—straight, lesbian, dominant/submissive and all sorts of extreme passions—are explored in thrilling detail.

STANLEY CARTEN
NAUGHTY MESSAGE
$5.95/333-3

Wesley Arthur discovers a lascivious message on his answering machine. Aroused beyond his wildest dreams by the acts described, Wesley becomes obsessed with tracking down the woman behind the seductive voice. His search takes him through strip clubs, sex parlors and no-tell motels—and finally to his randy reward....

MASQUERADE BOOKS

AKBAR DEL PIOMBO
SKIRTS
$4.95/115-2
Randy Mr. Edward Champdick enters high society—and a whole lot more—in his quest for ultimate satisfaction. For it seems that once Mr. Champdick rises to the occasion, nothing can bring him down.
DUKE COSIMO
$4.95/3052-0
A kinky romp played out against the boudoirs, bathrooms and ballrooms of the European nobility, who seem to do nothing all day except each other. The lifestyles of the rich and licentious are revealed in all their glory.
A CRUMBLING FAÇADE
$4.95/3043-1
The return of that incorrigible rogue, Henry Pike, who continues his pursuit of sex, fair or otherwise, in the most elegant homes of the most debauched aristocrats.

CAROLE REMY
BEAUTY OF THE BEAST
$5.95/332-5
A shocking tell-all, written from the point-of-view of a prize-winning reporter. And what reporting she does! All the secrets of an uninhibited life are revealed, and each lusty tableau is painted in glowing colors.

DAVID AARON CLARK
THE MARQUIS DE SADE'S JULIETTE
$4.95/240-X
The Marquis de Sade's infamous Juliette returns—and emerges as the most perverse and destructive nightstalker modern New York will ever know.

Praise for David Aaron Clark:

"David Aaron Clark has delved into one of the most sensationalistically taboo aspects of eros, sado-masochism, and produced a novel of unmistakable literary imagination and artistic value."
—Carlo McCormick, Paper

ANONYMOUS
NADIA
$5.95/267-1
Follow the delicious but neglected Nadia as she works to wring every drop of pleasure out of life—despite an unhappy marriage. A classic title providing a peek into the secret sexual lives of another time and place.

NIGEL McPARR
THE STORY OF A VICTORIAN MAID
$5.95/241-8
What were the Victorians really like? Chances are, no one believes they were as stuffy as their Queen, but who would have imagined such unbridled libertines! Follow her from exploit to smutty exploit!

MOLLY WEATHERFIELD
CARRIE'S STORY
$5.95/444-5
"I had been Jonathan's slave for about a year when he told me he wanted to sell me at an auction. I wasn't in any condition to respond when he told me this…." Desire and depravity run rampant in this story of uncompromising mastery and irrevocable submission.

BREN FLEMMING
CHARLY'S GAME
$4.95/221-3
A rich woman's gullible daughter has run off with one of the toughest leather dykes in town—and sexy P.I. Charly is hired to lure the girl back. One by one, wise and wicked women ensnare one another in their lusty nets!

ISADORA ALMAN
ASK ISADORA
$4.95/61-0
Six years' worth of Isadora Alman's syndicated columns on sex and relationships. Today's world is more perplexing than ever—and Alman can help untangle the most personal of knots.

TITIAN BERESFORD
THE WICKED HAND
$5.95/343-0
With an Introduction by Leg Show's Dian Hanson. A collection of fetishistic tales featuring the absolute subjugation of men by lovely, domineering women.
CINDERELLA
$6.50/500-X
Beresford triumphs again with this intoxicating tale, filled with castle dungeons and tightly corseted ladies-in-waiting, naughty viscounts and impossibly cruel masturbatrixes—nearly every conceivable method of erotic torture is explored and described in lush, vivid detail.
JUDITH BOSTON
$4.95/273-6
Young Edward would have been lucky to get the stodgy old companion he thought his parents had hired for him. Instead, an exquisite woman arrives at his door, and Edward finds his lewd behavior never goes unpunished by the unflinchingly severe Judith Boston! Together they take the downward path to perversion!
NINA FOXTON
$5.95/443-7
An aristocrat finds herself bored by run-of-the-mill amusements for "ladies of good breeding." Instead of taking tea with proper gentlemen, naughty Nina "milks" them of their most private essences. No man ever says "No" to the lovely Nina!

MASQUERADE BOOKS

A TITIAN BERESFORD READER
$4.95/114-4
Wild dominatrixes, perverse masochists, and mesmerizing detail are the hallmarks of the Beresford tale—and encountered here in abundance. The very best scenarios from all of Beresford's bestsellers.

P. N. DEDEAUX
THE NOTHING THINGS
$5.95/404-6
Beta Beta Rho—highly exclusive and widely honored—has taken on a new group of pledges. The five women will be put through the most grueling of ordeals, and punished severely for any shortcomings—much to everyone's delight!
TENDER BUNS
$5.95/396-1
In a fashionable Canadian suburb, Marc Merlin indulges his yen for punishment with an assortment of the town's most desirable and willing women. Things come to a rousing climax at a party planned to cater to just those whims Marc is most able to satisfy....

MICHAEL DRAX
OBSESSIONS
$4.95/3012-1
Victoria is determined to become a model by sexually ensnaring the powerful people who control the fashion industry: Paige, who finds herself compelled to watch Victoria's conquests; and Pietro and Alex, who take turns and then join in for a sizzling threesome. The story of one woman's unslakeable ambition—and lust!

LYN DAVENPORT
DOVER ISLAND
$5.95/384-8
Dr. David Kelly has planted the seeds of his dream—a Corporal Punishment Resort. Soon, many people from varied walks of life descend upon this isolated retreat, intent on fulfilling their every desire. Including Marcy Harris, the perfect partner for the lustful Doctor....
TESSA'S HOLIDAYS
$5.95/377-5
Tessa's lusty lover, Grant, makes sure that each of her holidays is filled with the type of sensual adventure most young women only dream about. What will he dream up next? Only he knows—and he keeps his secrets until the lovely Tessa is ready to explode with desire!
THE GUARDIAN
$5.95/371-6
Felicia grew up under the tutelage of the lash—and she learned her lessons well. Sir Rodney Wentworth has long searched for a woman capable of fulfilling his cruel desires, and after learning of Felicia's talents, sends for her. Felicia discovers that the "position" offered her is delightfully different than anything else she could have expected!

LIZBETH DUSSEAU
TRINKETS
$4.95/246-9
"Her bottom danced on the air, pert and fully round. It would take punishment well, he thought." A luscious woman submits to an artist's every whim—becoming the sexual trinket he had always desired.

ANTHONY BOBARZYNSKI
STASI SLUT
$4.95/3050-4
Adina lives in East Germany, where she meets a group of ruthless and corrupt STASI agents who use her for their own perverse gratification—until she uses her talents and attractions in a final bid for total freedom!

JOCELYN JOYCE
PRIVATE LIVES
$4.95/309-0
The lecherous habits of the illustrious make for a sizzling tale of French erotic life. A widow has a craving for a young busboy; he's sleeping with a rich businessman's wife; her husband is minding his sex business elsewhere! Scandalous sexual entanglements run through this tale of upper crust lust!
KIM'S PASSION
$4.95/162-4
The life of an insatiable seductress. Kim leaves India for London, where she quickly takes on the task of bedding every woman in sight!
CAROUSEL
$4.95/3051-2
A young American woman leaves her husband when she discovers he is having an affair with their maid. She then becomes the sexual plaything of Parisian voluptuaries.

SARAH JACKSON
SANCTUARY
$5.95/318-X
Sanctuary explores both the unspeakable debauchery of court life and the unimaginable privations of monastic solitude, leading the voracious and the virtuous on a collision course that brings history to throbbing life.
THE WILD HEART
$4.95/3007-5
A luxury hotel is the setting for this artful web of sex, desire, and love. A newlywed sees sex as a duty, while her hungry husband tries to awaken her to its tender joys. A Parisian entertains wealthy guests for the love of money. Each episode provides a new variation in this lusty Grand Hotel!

LOUISE BELHAVEL
FRAGRANT ABUSES
$4.95/88-2
The saga of Clara and Iris continues as the now-experienced girls enjoy themselves with a new circle of worldly friends whose imaginations match their own. Perversity follows the lusty ladies around the globe!

SARA H. FRENCH
MASTER OF TIMBERLAND
$5.95/327-9
A tale of sexual slavery at the ultimate paradise resort. One of our bestselling titles, this trek to Timberland has ignited passions the world over—and stands poised to become one of modern erotica's legendary tales.

MASQUERADE BOOKS

RETURN TO TIMBERLAND
$5.95/257-4
Prepare for a vacation filled with delicious decadence, as each and every visitor is serviced by unimaginably talented submissives. The raunchiest camp-out ever!

CHINA BLUE

KUNG FU NUNS
$4.95/3031-8
"She lifted me out of the chair and sat me down on top of the table. She then lifted her skirt. The sight of her perfect legs clad in white stockings and a petite garter belt further mesmerized me...." China Blue returns!

ROBERT DESMOND

THE SWEETEST FRUIT
$4.95/95-5
Connie is determined to seduce and destroy the devoted Father Chadcroft. She corrupts the unsuspecting priest into forsaking all that he holds sacred, and drags him into a hell of unbridled lust.

LUSCIDIA WALLACE

KATY'S AWAKENING
$4.95/308-2
Katy thinks she's been rescued after a terrible car wreck. Little does she suspect that she's been ensnared by a ring of swingers, whose tastes run to domination and unimaginably depraved sex parties. With no means of escape, Katy becomes the newest initiate in this sick private club—and soon finds herself becoming more depraved than even her degenerate captors.

MARY LOVE

MASTERING MARY SUE
$5.95/351-1
Mary Sue is a rich nymphomaniac whose husband is determined to declare her mentally incompetent and gain control of her fortune. He brings her to a castle where, to Mary Sue's delight, she is unleashed for a veritable sex-fest!

THE BEST OF MARY LOVE
$4.95/3099-7
Mary Love leaves no coupling untried and no extreme unexplored in these scandalous selections from *Mastering Mary Sue*, *Ecstasy on Fire*, *Vice Park Place*, *Wanda*, and *Naughtier at Night*.

AMARANTHA KNIGHT

THE DARKER PASSIONS: THE PICTURE OF DORIAN GRAY
$6.50/342-2
In this latest installment in the Darker Passions series, Amarantha Knight takes on Oscar Wilde, resulting in a fabulously decadent tale of highly personal changes. One young man finds his most secret desires laid bare by a portrait far more revealing than he could have imagined....

THE DARKER PASSIONS READER
$6.50/432-1
The best moments from Knight's phenomenally popular Darker Passions series. Here are the most eerily erotic passages from her acclaimed sexual reworkings of *Dracula*, *Frankenstein*, *Dr. Jekyll & Mr. Hyde* and *The Fall of the House of Usher*. Be prepared for more than a few thrills and chills from this arousing sampler.

THE DARKER PASSIONS: FRANKENSTEIN
$5.95/248-5
What if you could create a living human? What shocking acts could it be taught to perform, to desire? Find out what pleasures await those who play God....

THE DARKER PASSIONS: THE FALL OF THE HOUSE OF USHER
$5.95/313-9
The Master and Mistress of the house of Usher indulge in every form of decadence, and initiate their guests into the many pleasures to be found in utter submission.

THE DARKER PASSIONS: DR. JEKYLL AND MR. HYDE
$4.95/227-2
It is a story of incredible, frightening transformations achieved through mysterious experiments. Now, Amarantha Knight explores the steamy possibilities of a tale where no one is quite who—or what they seem. Victorian bedrooms explode with hidden demons!

THE DARKER PASSIONS: DRACULA
$5.95/326-0
The infamous erotic retelling of the Vampire legend. "Well-written and imaginative, Amarantha Knight gives fresh impetus to this myth, taking us through the sexual and sadistic scenes with details that keep us reading.... A classic in itself has been added to the shelves." —Divinity

PAUL LITTLE

THE BEST OF PAUL LITTLE
$6.50/469-0
One of Masquerade's all-time best-selling authors. Known throughout the world for his fantastic portrayals of punishment and pleasure, Little never fails to push readers over the edge of sensual excitement.

ALL THE WAY
$6.95/509-3
Two excruciating novels from Paul Little in one hot volume! *Going All the Way* features an unhappy man who tries to purge himself of the memory of his lover with a series of quirky and uninhibited lovers. *Pushover* tells the story of a serial spanker and his celebrated exploits.

THE DISCIPLINE OF ODETTE
$5.95/334-1
Odette's was sure marriage would rescue her from her family's "corrections." To her horror, she discovers that her beloved has also been raised on discipline. A shocking erotic coupling!

MASQUERADE BOOKS

THE PRISONER
$5.95/330-9
Judge Black has built a secret room below a penitentiary, where he sentences the prisoners to hours of exhibition and torment while his friends watch. Judge Black's House of Corrections is equipped with one purpose in mind: to administer his own brand of rough justice!

TEARS OF THE INQUISITION
$4.95/146-2
The incomparable Paul Little delivers a staggering account of pleasure and punishment. "There was a tickling inside her as her nervous system reminded her she was ready for sex. But before her was...the Inquisitor!"

DOUBLE NOVEL
$4.95/86-6
The Metamorphosis of Lisette Joyaux tells the story of a young woman initiated into a new world of lesbian lusts. *The Story of Monique* reveals the sexual rituals that beckon the ripe and willing Monique.

CHINESE JUSTICE AND OTHER STORIES
$4.95/153-5
The story of the excruciating pleasures and delicious punishments inflicted on foreigners under the leaders of the Boxer Rebellion. Each foreign woman is brought before the authorities and grilled. Scandalous deeds!

CAPTIVE MAIDENS
$5.95/440-2
Three beautiful young women find themselves powerless against the debauched landowners of 1824 England. They are banished to a sexual slave colony, and corrupted by every imaginable perversion. Soon, they come to crave the treatment of their unrelenting captors, and find themselves insatiable.

SLAVE ISLAND
$5.95/441-0
A leisure cruise is waylaid, finding itself in the domain of Lord Henry Philbrock, a sadistic genius. The ship's passengers are kidnapped and spirited to his island prison, where the women are trained to accommodate the most bizarre sexual cravings of the rich, the famous, the pampered and the perverted. An incredible bestseller, which cemented Little's reputation as a master of contemporary erotic literature.

ALIZARIN LAKE
SEX ON DOCTOR'S ORDERS
$5.95/402-X
A chronicle of selfless devotion to mankind! Beth, a nubile young nurse, uses her considerable skills to further medical science by offering incomparable and insatiable assistance in the gathering of important specimens. No man leaves naughty Nurse Beth's station without surrendering exactly what she needs!

THE EROTIC ADVENTURES OF HARRY TEMPLE
$4.95/127-6
Harry Temple's memoirs chronicle his amorous adventures from his initiation at the hands of insatiable sirens, through his stay at a house of hot repute, to his encounters with a chastity-belted nympho!

JOHN NORMAN
TARNSMAN OF GOR
$6.95/486-0
This legendary—and controversial—series returns! *Tarnsman* finds Tarl Cabot transported to Counter-Earth, better known as Gor. He must quickly accustom himself to the ways of this world, including the caste system which exalts some as Priest-Kings or Warriors, and debases others as slaves. A spectacular world unfolds in this first volume of John Norman's million-selling Gorean series.

OUTLAW OF GOR
$6.95/487-9
In this second volume, Tarl Cabot returns to Gor, where he might reclaim both his woman and his role of Warrior. But upon arriving, he discovers that his name, his city and the names of those he loves have become unspeakable. In his absence, Cabot has become an outlaw, and must discover his new purpose on this strange planet, where danger stalks the outcast, and even simple answers have their price....

PRIEST-KINGS OF GOR
$6.95/488-7
The third volume of John Norman's million-selling, controversial Gor series. Tarl Cabot, brave Tarnsman of Gor, searches for the truth about his lovely wife Talena. Does she live, or was she destroyed by the mysterious, all-powerful Priest-Kings? Cabot is determined to find out— while knowing that no one who has approached the mountain stronghold of the Priest-Kings has ever returned alive....

RACHEL PEREZ
ODD WOMEN
$4.95/123-3
These women are sexy, smart, tough—some even say odd. But who cares, when their combined ass-ets are so sweet! An assortment of Sapphic sirens proves once and for all that comely ladies come best in pairs.

ALIZARIN LAKE
SEX ON DOCTOR'S ORDERS
$5.95/402-X
Beth, a nubile young nurse, uses her considerable skills to further medical science by offering incomparable and insatiable assistance in the gathering of important specimens. No man leaves naughty Nurse Beth's station without surrendering exactly what she needs!

THE EROTIC ADVENTURES OF HARRY TEMPLE
$4.95/127-6
Harry Temple's memoirs chronicle his amorous adventures from his initiation at the hands of insatiable sirens, through his stay at a house of hot repute, to his encounters with a chastity-belted nympho!

AFFINITIES
$4.95/113-6
"Kelsy had a liking for cool upper-class blondes, the long-legged girls from Lake Forest and Winnetka who came into the city to cruise the lesbian bars on Halsted, looking for breathless ecstasies...." A scorching tale of lesbian libidos unleashed, from a writer more than capable of exploring every nuance of female passion in vivid detail.

MASQUERADE BOOKS

SYDNEY ST. JAMES

RIVE GAUCHE
$5.95/317-1
The Latin Quarter, Paris, circa 1920. Expatriate bohemians couple with abandon—before eventually abandoning their ambitions amidst the intoxicating temptations waiting to be indulged in every bedroom.

THE HIGHWAYWOMAN
$4.95/174-8
A young filmmaker making a documentary about the life of the notorious English highwaywoman, Bess Ambrose, becomes obsessed with her mysterious subject. It seems that Bess touched more than hearts—and plundered the treasures of every man and maiden she met on the way. Incredible extremes of passion are reached by not only the voluptuous filmmaker, but her insatiable subject!

GARDEN OF DELIGHT
$4.95/3058-X
A vivid account of sexual awakening that follows an innocent but insatiably curious young woman's journey from the furtive, forbidden joys of dormitory life to the unabashed carnality of the wild world. A coming of age story unlike any other!

MARCUS VAN HELLER

TERROR
$5.95/247-7
Another shocking exploration of lust by the author of the ever-popular *Adam & Eve*. Set in Paris during the Algerian War, Terror explores the place of sexual passion in a world drunk on violence.

KIDNAP
$4.95/90-4
P. I. Harding is called in to investigate a mysterious kidnapping case involving the rich and powerful. Along the way he has the pleasure of "interrogating" an exotic dancer named Jeanne and a beautiful English reporter, as he finds himself enmeshed in the crime underworld.

ALEXANDER TROCCHI

THONGS
$4.95/217-5
"...In Spain, life is cheap, from that glittering tragedy in the bullring to the quick thrust of the stiletto in a narrow street in a Barcelona slum. No, this death would not have called for further comment had it not been for one striking fact. The naked woman had met her end in a way he had never seen before—a way that had enormous sexual significance. My God, she had been..." Trocchi's acclaimed classic returns.

HELEN AND DESIRE
$4.95/3093-8
Helen Seferis' flight from the oppressive village of her birth became a sexual tour of a harsh world. From brothels in Sydney to harems in Algiers, Helen chronicles her adventures fully in her diary. Each encounter is examined in the scorching and uncensored diary of the sensual Helen!

THE CARNAL DAYS OF HELEN SEFERIS
$4.95/3086-5
P.I. Anthony Harvest is assigned to save Helen Seferis, a beautiful Australian who has been abducted. Following clues in her explicit diary of adventures, he pursues the lovely, doomed Helen—the ultimate sexual prize.

DON WINSLOW

THE INSATIABLE MISTRESS OF ROSEDALE
$6.50/494-1
The story of the perfect couple: Edward and Lady Penelope, who reside in beautiful and mysterious Rosedale manor. While Edward is a true connoisseur of sexual perversion, it is Lady Penelope whose mastery of complete sensual pleasure makes their home infamous. Indulging one another's bizarre whims is a way of life for this wicked couple, and none who encounter the extravagances of Rosedale will forget what they've learned....

SECRETS OF CHEATEM MANOR
$6.50/434-8
Edward returns to his late father's estate, to find it being run by the majestic Lady Amanda. Edward can hardly believe his luck—Lady Amanda is assisted by her two beautiful, lonely daughters, Catherine and Prudence. What the randy young man soon comes to realize is the love of discipline that all three beauties share.

KATERINA IN CHARGE
$5.95/409-7
When invited to a country retreat by a mysterious couple, the two randy young ladies can hardly resist! But do they have any idea what they're in for? Whatever the case, the imperious Katerina will make her desires known very soon—and demand that they be fulfilled...

THE MANY PLEASURES OF IRONWOOD
$5.95/310-4
Seven lovely young women are employed by The Ironwood Sportsmen's Club A small and exclusive club with seven carefully selected sexual connoisseurs, Ironwood is dedicated to the relentless pursuit of sensual pleasure.

CLAIRE'S GIRLS
$5.95/442-9
You knew when she walked by that she was something special. She was one of Claire's girls, a woman carefully dressed and groomed to fill a role, to capture a look, to fit an image crafted by the sophisticated proprietress of an exclusive escort agency. High-class whores blow the roof off!

N. WHALLEN

TAU'TEVU
$6.50/426-7
In a mysterious land, the statuesque and beautiful Vivian learns to subject herself to the hand of a mysterious man. He systematically helps her prove her own strength, and brings to life in her an unimagined sensual fire. But who is this man, who goes only by the name of Orpheo?

BUY ANY 4 BOOKS & CHOOSE 1 ADDITIONAL BOOK, OF EQUAL OR LESSER VALUE, AS YOUR FREE GIFT

MASQUERADE BOOKS

COMPLIANCE
$5.95/356-2

Fourteen stories exploring the pleasures of release. Characters from all walks of life learn to trust in the skills of others, only to experience the thrilling liberation of submission. Here are the joys to be found in some of the most forbidden sexual practices around....

THE MASQUERADE READERS

THE VELVET TONGUE
$4.95/3029-6

An orgy of oral gratification! The Velvet Tongue celebrates the most mouth-watering, lip-smacking, tongue-twisting action. A feast of fellatio and soixante-neuf awaits readers of excellent taste at this steamy suck-fest.

A MASQUERADE READER
$4.95/84-X

A sizzling sampler. Strict lessons are learned at the hand of The English Governess. Scandalous confessions are found in The Diary of an Angel, and the story of a woman whose desires drove her to the ultimate sacrifice in Thongs completes the collection.

THE CLASSIC COLLECTION

PROTESTS, PLEASURES, RAPTURES
$5.95/400-3

Invited for an allegedly quiet weekend at a country vicarage, a young woman is stunned to find herself surrounded by shocking acts of sexual sadism. Soon, her curiosity is piqued, and she begins to explore her own capacities for cruelty.

THE YELLOW ROOM
$5.95/378-3

The "yellow room" holds the secrets of lust, lechery, and the lash. There, bare-bottomed, spread-eagled, and open to the world, demure Alice Darvell soon learns to love her lickings. In the second tale, hot heiress Rosa Coote and her adventures in punishment and pleasure.

SCHOOL DAYS IN PARIS
$5.95/325-2

The rapturous chronicles of a well-spent youth! Few Universities provide the profound and pleasurable lessons one learns in after-hours study—particularly if one is young and available, and lucky enough to have Paris as a playground. A stimulating look at the pursuits of young adulthood.

MAN WITH A MAID
$4.95/307-4

The adventures of Jack and Alice have delighted readers for eight decades! A classic of its genre, Man with a Maid tells an outrageous tale of desire, revenge, and submission. This tale qualifies as one of the world's most popular adult novels—with over 200,000 copies in print!

MAN WITH A MAID II
$4.95/3071-7

Jack's back! With the assistance of the perverse Alice, he embarks again on a trip through every erotic extreme. Jack leaves no one unsatisfied—least of all, himself—and Alice is always certain to outdo herself in her capacity to corrupt and control. An incendiary sequel!

MAN WITH A MAID: THE CONCLUSION
$4.95/3013-X

The conclusion to the epic saga of lust that has thrilled readers for decades. The adulterous woman who is corrected with enthusiasm and the maid who receives grueling guidance are just two who benefit from these lessons!

CONFESSIONS OF A CONCUBINE III: PLEASURE'S PRISONER
$5.95/357-0

Filled with pulse-pounding excitement—including a daring escape from the harem and an encounter with an unspeakable sadist—Pleasure's Prisoner adds an unforgettable chapter to this thrilling confessional.

CONFESSIONS OF A CONCUBINE II: HAREM SLAVE
$4.95/226-4

The concubinage continues, as the true pleasures and privileges of the harem are revealed. For the first time, readers are invited behind the veils that hide uninhibited, unimaginable pleasures from the world....

LADY F.
$4.95/102-0

An uncensored tale of Victorian passions. Master Kidrodstock suffers deliciously at the hands of the stunningly cruel and sensuous Lady Flayskin—the only woman capable of taming his wayward impulses. A fevered chronicle of punishing passions.

CLASSIC EROTIC BIOGRAPHIES

JENNIFER III
$5.95/292-2

The further adventures of erotica's most daring heroine. Jennifer, the quintessential beautiful blonde, has a photographer's eye for details—particularly of the masculine variety!

JENNIFER AGAIN
$4.95/220-5

One of modern erotica's most famous heroines. Once again, the insatiable Jennifer seizes the day—and extracts from it every last drop of sensual pleasure! No man is immune to this vixen's charms.

JENNIFER
$4.95/107-1

From the bedroom of a notoriously insatiable dancer to an uninhibited ashram, Jennifer traces the exploits of one thoroughly modern woman as she lustfully explores the limits of her own sexuality.

THE ROMANCES OF BLANCHE LA MARE
$4.95/101-2

When Blanche loses her husband, it becomes clear she'll need a job. She sets her sights on the stage—and soon encounters a cast of lecherous characters intent on making her path to sucksess as hot and hard as possible!

PETER JASON

WAYWARD
$4.95/3004-0

A mysterious countess hires a tour bus for an unusual vacation. Traveling through Europe's most notorious cities, she picks up friends, lovers, and acquaintances from every walk of life in pursuit of pleasure.

MASQUERADE BOOKS

ROMY ROSEN

SPUNK
$6.95/492-5

A scintillating tale of unearthly beauty, outrageous decadence, and brutal exploitation. Casey, a lovely model poised upon the verge of super-celebrity, falls hard for a insatiable young rock singer—not suspecting that his sexual appetite has led him to experiment with a dangerous new aphrodisiac. Casey becomes an addict, and her craving plunges her into a strange underworld, where bizarre sexual compulsions are indulged behind the most exclusive doors and the only chance for redemption lies with a shadowy young man with a secret of his own.

CYBERSEX CONSORTIUM

THE PERV'S GUIDE TO THE INTERNET
$6.95/471-1

You've heard the objections: cyberspace is soaked with sex, piled high with prurience, mired in immorality. Okay—so where is it!? Tracking down the good stuff—the real good stuff—can waste an awful lot of expensive time, and frequently leave you high and dry. But now, the Cybersex Consortium presents an easy-to-use guide for those intrepid adults who know what they want. No horny hacker can afford to pass up this map to the kinkiest rest stops on the Info Superhighway.

AMELIA G, EDITOR

BACKSTAGE PASSES
$6.96/438-0

A collection of some of the most raucous writing around. Amelia G, editor of the goth-sex journal *Blue Blood*, has brought together some of today's most irreverant writers, each of whom has outdone themselves with an edgy, antic tale of modern lust. Punks, metalheads, and grunge-trash roam the pages of *Backstage Passes*, and no one knows their ways better...

GERI NETTICK WITH BETH ELLIOT

MIRRORS: PORTRAIT OF A LESBIAN TRANSSEXUAL
$6.95/435-6

The alternately heartbreaking and empowering story of one woman's long road to full selfhood. Born a male, Geri Nettick knew something just didn't fit. And even after coming to terms with her own gender dysphoria—and taking steps to correct it—she still fought to be accepted by the lesbian feminist community to which she felt she belonged. A fascinating, true tale of struggle and discovery.

TRISTAN TAORMINO & DAVID AARON CLARK, EDITORS

RITUAL SEX
$6.95/391-0

While many people believe the body and soul to occupy almost completely independent realms, the many contributors to *Ritual Sex* know—and demonstrate—that the two share more common ground than society feels comfortable acknowledging. From personal memoirs of ecstatic revelation, to fictional quests to reconcile sex and spirit, *Ritual Sex* delves into forbidden areas with gusto, providing an unprecedented look at private life.

DAVID MELTZER

UNDER
$6.95/290-6

The story of a sex professional living at the bottom of the social heap. After surgeries designed to increase his physical allure, corrupt government forces drive the cyber-gigolo underground—where even more bizarre cultures await him.

ORF
$6.95/110-1

He is the ultimate musician-hero—the idol of thousands, the fevered dream of many more. And like many musicians before him, he is misunderstood, misused—and totally out of control. Every last drop of feeling is squeezed from a modern-day troubadour and his lady love.

TAMMY JO ECKHART

PUNISHMENT FOR THE CRIME
$6.95/427-5

Peopled by characters of rare depth, these stories explore the true meaning of dominance and submission, and offer some surprising revelations. From an encounter between two of society's most despised individuals, to the explorations of longtime friends, these tales take you where few others have ever dared....

THOMAS S. ROCHE, EDITOR

NOIROTICA: AN ANTH. OF EROTIC CRIME STORIES
$6.95/390-2

A collection of darkly sexy tales, taking place at the crossroads of the crime and erotic genres. Thomas S. Roche has gathered together some of today's finest writers of sexual fiction, all of whom explore the murky terrain where desire runs irrevocably afoul of the law.

AMARANTHA KNIGHT, EDITOR

SEDUCTIVE SPECTRES
$6.95/464-X

Breathtaking tours through the erotic supernatural via the macabre imaginations of today's best writers. Never before have ghostly encounters been so alluring, thanks to a cast of otherworldly characters well-acquainted with the pleasures of the flesh.

MASQUERADE BOOKS

SEX MACABRE
$6.95/392-9

Horror tales designed for dark and sexy nights. Amarantha Knight—the woman behind the Darker Passions series, as well as the spine-tingling anthologies *Flesh Fantastic* and *Love Bites*—has gathered together erotic stories sure to make your skin crawl, and heart beat faster.

FLESH FANTASTIC
$6.95/352-X

Humans have long toyed with the idea of "playing God": creating life from nothingness, bringing life to the inanimate. Now Amarantha Knight, author of the "Darker Passions" series, collects stories exploring not only the act of Creation, but the lust that follows....

GARY BOWEN

DIARY OF A VAMPIRE
$6.95/331-7

"Gifted with a darkly sensual vision and a fresh voice, [Bowen] is a writer to watch out for."

—Cecilia Tan

The chilling, arousing, and ultimately moving memoirs of an undead—but all too human—soul. Bowen's Rafael, a red-blooded male with an insatiable hunger for the same, is the perfect antidote to the effete malcontents haunting bookstores today. *Diary of a Vampire* marks the emergence of a bold and brilliant vision, firmly rooted in past and present.

LAURA ANTONIOU, EDITOR

NO OTHER TRIBUTE
$6.95/294-9

A collection sure to challenge Political Correctness in a way few have before, with tales of women kept in bondage to their lovers by their deepest passions. Love pushes these women beyond acceptable limits, rendering them helpless to deny anything to the men and women they adore. A volume dedicated to all Slaves of Desire.

SOME WOMEN
$6.95/300-7

Over forty essays written by women actively involved in consensual dominance and submission. Professional mistresses, lifestyle leatherdykes, whipmakers, titleholders—women from every conceivable walk of life lay bare their true feelings about explosive issues.

BY HER SUBDUED
$6.95/281-7

These tales all involve women in control—of their lives, their loves, their men. So much in control that they can remorselessly break rules to become powerful goddesses of the men who sacrifice all to worship at their feet.

RENÉ MAIZEROY

FLESHLY ATTRACTIONS
$6.95/299-X

Lucien was the son of the wantonly beautiful actress, Marie-Rose Hardanges. When she decides to let a "friend" introduce her son to the pleasures of love, Marie-Rose could not have foretold the excesses that would lead to her own ruin and that of her cherished son.

JEAN STINE

THRILL CITY
$6.95/411-9

Thrill City is the seat of the world's increasing depravity, and Jean Stine's classic novel transports you there with a vivid style you'd be hard pressed to ignore. No writer is better suited to describe the unspeakable extremes of this modern Babylon.

SEASON OF THE WITCH
$6.95/268-X

"A future in which it is technically possible to transfer the total mind...of a rapist killer into the brain dead but physically living body of his female victim. Remarkable for intense psychological technique. There is eroticism but it is necessary to mark the differences between the sexes and the subtle altering of a man into a woman."

—*The Science Fiction Critic*

JOHN WARREN

THE TORQUEMADA KILLER
$6.95/367-8

Detective Eva Hernandez gets her first "big case": a string of vicious murders taking place within New York's SM community. Eva assembles the evidence, revealing a picture of a world misunderstood and under attack—and gradually comes to understand her own place within it.

THE LOVING DOMINANT
$6.95/218-3

Everything you need to know about an infamous sexual variation—and an unspoken type of love. Mentor—a longtime player in scene—guides readers through this world and reveals the too-often hidden basis of the D/S relationship: care, trust and love.

GRANT ANTREWS

MY DARLING DOMINATRIX
$6.95/447-X

When a man and a woman fall in love, it's supposed to be simple, uncomplicated, easy—unless that woman happens to be a dominatrix. Curiosity gives way to unblushing desire in this story of one man's awakening to the joys of willing slavery.

LAURA ANTONIOU WRITING AS "SARA ADAMSON"

THE TRAINER
$6.95/249-3

The Marketplace—the ultimate underground sexual realm includes not only willing slaves, but the exquisite trainers who take submissives firmly in hand. And now these mentors divulge the desires that led them to become the ultimate figures of authority.

THE SLAVE
$6.95/173-X

This second volume in the "Marketplace" trilogy further elaborates the world of slaves and masters. One talented submissive longs to join the ranks of those who have proven themselves worthy of entry into the Marketplace. But the delicious price is staggeringly high....

MASQUERADE BOOKS

THE MARKETPLACE
$6.95/3096-2
"Merchandise does not come easily to the Marketplace.... They haunt the clubs and the organizations.... Some are so ripe that they intimidate the poseurs, the weekend sadists and the furtive dilettantes who are so endemic to that world. And they never stop asking where we may be found...."

DAVID AARON CLARK
SISTER RADIANCE
$6.95/215-9
Rife with Clark's trademark vivisections of contemporary desires, sacred and profane. The vicissitudes of lust and romance are examined against a backdrop of urban decay in this testament to the allure of the forbidden.
THE WET FOREVER
$6.95/117-9
The story of Janus and Madchen—a small-time hood and a beautiful sex worker on the run from one of the most dangerous men they have ever known—The Wet Forever examines themes of loyalty, sacrifice, redemption and obsession amidst Manhattan's sex parlors and underground S/M clubs. Its combination of sex and suspense led Terence Sellers to proclaim it "evocative and poetic."

MICHAEL PERKINS
EVIL COMPANIONS
$6.95/3067-9
Set in New York City during the tumultuous waning years of the Sixties, Evil Companions has been hailed as "a frightening classic." A young couple explores the nether reaches of the erotic unconscious in a shocking confrontation with the extremes of passion.
THE SECRET RECORD: MODERN EROTIC LITERATURE
$6.95/3039-3
Michael Perkins surveys the field with authority and unique insight. Updated and revised to include the latest trends, tastes, and developments in this misunderstood and maligned genre.
AN ANTHOLOGY OF CLASSIC ANONYMOUS EROTIC WRITING
$6.95/140-3
Michael Perkins has collected the very best passages from the world's erotic writing. "Anonymous" is one of the most infamous bylines in publishing history—and these steamy excerpts show why! Includes excerpts from some of the most famous titles in the history of erotic literature.

LIESEL KULIG
LOVE IN WARTIME
$6.95/3044-X
Madeleine knew that the handsome SS officer was a dangerous man, but he was just a cabaret singer in Nazi-occupied Paris, trying to survive in a perilous time. When Josef fell in love with her, he discovered that a beautiful and amoral woman can sometimes be wildly dangerous.

HELEN HENLEY
ENTER WITH TRUMPETS
$6.95/197-7
Helen Henley was told that women just don't write about sex—much less the taboos she was so interested in exploring. So Henley did it alone, flying in the face of "tradition," by writing this touching tale of arousal and devotion in one couple's kinky relationship.

ALICE JOANOU
BLACK TONGUE
$6.95/258-2
"Joanou has created a series of sumptuous, brooding, dark visions of sexual obsession, and is undoubtedly a name to look out for in the future."
—Redeemer
Exploring lust at its most florid and unsparing, Black Tongue is a trove of baroque fantasies—each redolent of forbidden passions. Joanou creates some of erotica's most mesmerizing and unforgettable characters.
TOURNIQUET
$6.95/3060-1
A heady collection of stories and effusions from the pen of one our most dazzling young writers. Strange tales abound, from the story of the mysterious and cruel Cybele, to an encounter with the sadistic entertainment of a bizarre after-hours cafe. A complex and riveting series of meditations on desire.
CANNIBAL FLOWER
$4.95/72-6
The provocative debut volume from this acclaimed writer. "She is waiting in her darkened bedroom, as she has waited throughout history, to seduce the men who are foolish enough to be blinded by her irresistible charms.... She is the goddess of sexuality, and Cannibal Flower is her haunting siren song."
—Michael Perkins

TUPPY OWENS
SENSATIONS
$6.95/3081-4
Tuppy Owens tells the unexpurgated story of the making of Sensations—the first big-budget sex flick. Originally commissioned to appear in book form after the release of the film in 1975, Sensations is finally released under Masquerade's stylish Rhinoceros imprint.

SOPHIE GALLEYMORE BIRD
MANEATER
$6.95/103-9
Through a bizarre act of creation, a man attains the "perfect" lover—by all appearances a beautiful, sensuous woman, but in reality something far darker. Once brought to life she will accept no mate, seeking instead the prey that will sate her hunger for vengeance. A biting take on the war of the sexes, this debut goes for the jugular of the "perfect woman" myth.

MASQUERADE BOOKS

PHILIP JOSÉ FARMER

FLESH
$6.95/303-1
Space Commander Stagg explored the galaxies for 800 years. Upon his return, Stagg is made the centerpiece of an incredible public ritual—one that will repeatedly take him to the heights of ecstasy, and inexorably drag him toward the depths of hell.

A FEAST UNKNOWN
$6.95/276-0
"Sprawling, brawling, shocking, suspenseful, hilarious..."
—Theodore Sturgeon
Farmer's supreme anti-hero returns. "I was conceived and born in 1888." Slowly, Lord Grandrith—armed with the belief that he is the son of Jack the Ripper—tells the story of his remarkable and unbridled life. His story begins with his discovery of the secret of immortality—and progresses to encompass the furthest extremes of human behavior. A classic of speculative erotica.

THE IMAGE OF THE BEAST
$6.95/166-7
Herald Childe has seen Hell, glimpsed its horror in an act of sexual mutilation. Childe must now find and destroy an inhuman predator through the streets of a polluted and decadent Los Angeles of the future. One clue after another leads Childe to an inescapable realization about the nature of sex and evil....

DANIEL VIAN

ILLUSIONS
$6.95/3074-1
Two tales of danger and desire in Berlin on the eve of WWII. From private homes to lurid cafés, passion is exposed in stark contrast to the brutal violence of the time. Two sexy tales examining a remarkably decadent age.

PERSUASIONS
$6.95/183-7
A double novel, including the classics *Adagio* and *Gabriela and the General*, this volume traces desire around the globe. Two classics of international lust!

SAMUEL R. DELANY

THE MAD MAN
$8.99/408-9
"Reads like a pornographic reflection of Peter Ackroyd's *Chatterton* or A. S. Byatt's *Possession*.... Delany develops an insightful dichotomy between [his protagonist]'s two worlds: the one of cerebral philosophy and dry academia, the other of heedless, 'impersonal' obsessive sexual extremism. When these worlds finally collide...the novel achieves a surprisingly satisfying resolution...."
—*Publishers Weekly*
For his thesis, graduate student John Marr researches the life of Timothy Hasler: a philosopher whose career was cut tragically short over a decade earlier. On another front, Marr finds himself increasingly drawn toward shocking, depraved sexual entanglements with the homeless men of his neighborhood, until it begins to seem that Hasler's death might hold some key to his own life as a gay man in the age of AIDS.

EQUINOX
$6.95/157-8
The Scorpion has sailed the seas in a quest for every possible pleasure. Her crew is a collection of the young, the twisted, the insatiable. A drifter comes into their midst and is taken on a fantastic journey to the darkest, most dangerous sexual extremes—until he is finally a victim to their boundless appetites.

ANDREI CODRESCU
THE REPENTANCE OF LORRAINE
$6.95/329-5
"One of our most prodigiously talented and magical writers."
—*NYT Book Review*
By the acclaimed author of *The Hole in the Flag* and *The Blood Countess*. An aspiring writer, a professor's wife, a secretary, gold anklets, Maoists, Roman harlots—and more—swirl through this spicy tale of a harried quest for a mythic artifact. Written when the author was a young man, this lusty yarn was inspired by the heady days of the Sixties.

LEOPOLD VON SACHER-MASOCH
VENUS IN FURS
$6.95/3089-X
This classic 19th century novel is the first uncompromising exploration of the dominant/submissive relationship in literature. The alliance of Severin and Wanda epitomizes Sacher-Masoch's dark obsession with a cruel, controlling goddess and the urges that drive the man held in her thrall. This special edition includes the letters exchanged between Sacher-Masoch and Emilie Mataja, an aspiring writer he sought to cast as the avatar of the forbidden desires expressed in his most famous work.

BADBOY

JULIAN ANTHONY GUERRA, EDITOR
COME QUICKLY: FOR BOYS ON THE GO
$6.50/413-5
The increasing pace of daily life is no reason a guy has to forgo a little carnal pleasure whenever the mood strikes him. Here are over sixty of the hottest fantasies around—all designed to get you going in less time than it takes to dial 976. Julian Anthony Guerra, the editor behind the phenomenally popular *Men at Work* and *Badboy Fantasies*, has put together this volume especially for you—a man on a modern schedule, who still appreciates a little old-fashioned action.

MATT TOWNSEND
SOLIDLY BUILT
$6.50/416-X
The tale of the tumultuous relationship between Jeff, a young photographer, and Mark, the butch electrician hired to wire Jeff's new home. For Jeff, it's love at first sight; Mark, however, has more than a few hang-ups. Soon, both are forced to reevaluate their outlooks, and are assisted by a variety of hot men....

MASQUERADE BOOKS

JOHN PRESTON

MR. BENSON
$4.95/3041-5
A classic erotic novel from a time when there was no limit to what a man could dream of doing.... Jamie is an aimless young man lucky enough to encounter Mr. Benson. He is soon led down the path of erotic enlightenment, learning to accept this man as his master. Jamie's incredible adventures never fail to excite—especially when the going gets rough!

TALES FROM THE DARK LORD
$5.95/323-6
A new collection of twelve stunning works from the man *Lambda Book Report* called "the Dark Lord of gay erotica." The relentless ritual of lust and surrender is explored in all its manifestations in this heart-stopping triumph of authority and vision from the Dark Lord!

TALES FROM THE DARK LORD II
$4.95/176-4
The second volume of acclaimed eroticist John Preston's masterful short stories. Also includes an interview with the author, and an explicit screenplay written for pornstar Scott O'Hara.

THE ARENA
$4.95/3083-0
There is a place on the edge of fantasy where every desire is indulged with abandon. Men go there to unleash beasts, to let demons roam free, to abolish all limits. At the center of each tale are the men who serve there, who offer themselves for the consummation of any passion, whose own bottomless urges compel their endless subservience.

THE HEIR•THE KING
$4.95/3048-2
The ground-breaking novel *The Heir*, written in the lyric voice of the ancient myths, tells the story of a world where slaves and masters create a new sexual society. This edition also includes a completely original work, *The King*, the story of a soldier who discovers his monarch's most secret desires. Available only from Badboy.

THE MISSION OF ALEX KANE

SWEET DREAMS
$4.95/3062-8
It's the triumphant return of gay action hero Alex Kane! In *Sweet Dreams*, Alex travels to Boston where he takes on a street gang that stalks gay teenagers. Mighty Alex Kane wreaks a fierce and terrible vengeance on those who prey on gay people everywhere!

GOLDEN YEARS
$4.95/3069-5
When evil threatens the plans of a group of older gay men, Kane's got the muscle to take it head on. Along the way, he wins the support—and very specialized attentions—of a cowboy plucked right out of the Old West. But Kane and the Cowboy have a surprise waiting for them....

DEADLY LIES
$4.95/3076-8
Politics is a dirty business and the dirt becomes deadly when a political smear campaign targets gay men. Who better to clean things up than Alex Kane! Alex comes to protect the dreams, and lives, of gay men imperiled by lies.

STOLEN MOMENTS
$4.95/3098-9
Houston's evolving gay community is victimized by a malicious newspaper editor who is more than willing to sacrifice gays on the altar of circulation. He never counted on Alex Kane, fearless defender of gay dreams and desires.

SECRET DANGER
$4.95/111-X
Homophobia: a pernicious social ill not confined by America's borders. Alex Kane and the faithful Danny are called to a small European country, where a group of gay tourists is being held hostage by ruthless terrorists. Luckily, the Mission of Alex Kane stands as firm foreign policy.

LETHAL SILENCE
$4.95/125-X
The Mission of Alex Kane thunders to a conclusion. Chicago becomes the scene of the right-wing's most noxious plan—facilitated by unholy political alliances. Alex and Danny head to the Windy City to take up battle with the mercenaries who would squash gay men underfoot.

JAY SHAFFER

WET DREAMS
$6.50/495-X
Sweaty, sloppy sex runs throughout this collection of superhot, hypermasculine sex-tales from one of our most accomplished Badboys. Each of these stories takes a hot, hard look at the obsessions that keep men up all night. Provocative and affecting, this is a night full of dreams you won't forget in the morning.

SHOOTERS
$5.95/284-1
No mere catalog of random acts, *Shooters* tells the stories of a variety of stunning men and the ways they connect in sexual and non-sexual ways. A virtuoso storyteller, Shaffer always gets his man.

ANIMAL HANDLERS
$4.95/264-7
In Shaffer's world, each and every man finally succumbs to the animal urges deep inside. And if there's any creature that promises a wild time, it's a beast who's been caged for far too long.

FULL SERVICE
$4.95/150-0
Wild men build up steam until they finally let loose. Nononsense guys bear down hard on each other as they work their way toward release in this finely detailed assortment of masculine fantasies. One of gay erotica's most insightful chroniclers of male passion.

MASQUERADE BOOKS

D. V. SADERO

REVOLT OF THE NAKED
$4.95/261-2
In a distant galaxy, there are two classes of humans: Freemen and Nakeds. Freemen are full citizens; Nakeds live only to serve their Masters, and obey every sexual order with haste and devotion.

IN THE ALLEY
$4.95/144-6
Hardworking men—from cops to carpenters—bring their own special skills and impressive tools to the most satisfying job of all: capturing and breaking the male sexual beast. Hot, incisive and way over the top!

SCOTT O'HARA

DO-IT-YOURSELF PISTON POLISHING
$6.50/489-5
Longtime sex-pro Scott O'Hara draws upon his acute powers of seduction to lure you into a world of hard, horny men long overdue for a tune-up. Pretty soon, you'll pop your own hood for the servicing you know you need....

SUTTER POWELL

EXECUTIVE PRIVILEGES
$6.50/383-X
No matter how serious or sexy a predicament his characters find themselves in, Powell conveys the sheer exuberance of their encounters with a warm humor rarely seen in contemporary gay erotica.

GARY BOWEN

MAN HUNGRY
$5.95/374-0
By the author of Diary of a Vampire. A riveting collection of stories from one of gay erotica's new stars. Dipping into a variety of genres, Bowen crafts tales of lust unlike anything being published today.

KYLE STONE

FIRE & ICE
$5.95/297-3
A collection of stories from the author of the infamous adventures of PB 500. Randy, powerful, and just plain bad, Stone's characters always promise one thing: enough hot action to burn away your desire for anyone else....

HOT BAUDS
$5.95/285-X
The author of Fantasy Board and The Initiation of PB 500 combed cyberspace for the hottest fantasies of the world's horniest hackers. Stone has assembled the first collection of the raunchy erotica so many gay men cruise the Information Superhighway for.

FANTASY BOARD
$4.95/212-4
The author of the scalding sci-fi adventures of PB 500 explores the more foreseeable future—through the intertwined lives (and private parts) of a collection of randy computer hackers. On the Lambda Gate BBS, every hot and horny male is in search of a little virtual satisfaction.

THE CITADEL
$4.95/198-5
The sequel to The Initiation of PB 500. Having proven himself worthy of his stunning master, Micah—now known only as '500'—will face new challenges and hardships after his entry into the forbidding Citadel. Only his master knows what awaits—and whether Micah will again distinguish himself as the perfect instrument of pleasure....

THE INITIATION OF PB 500
$4.95/141-1
An interstellar accident strands a young stud on an alien planet. He is a stranger on their planet, unschooled in their language, and ignorant of their customs. But this man, Micah—now known only by his number—will soon be trained in every last detail of erotic personal service. And, once nurtured and transformed into the perfect physical specimen, he must begin proving himself worthy of the master who has chosen him....

RITUALS
$4.95/168-3
Via a computer bulletin board, a young man finds himself drawn into a series of sexual rites that transform him into the willing slave of a mysterious stranger. Gradually, all vestiges of his former life are thrown off, and he learns to live for his Master's touch....

JOHN ROWBERRY

LEWD CONDUCT
$4.95/3091-1
Flesh-and-blood men vie for power, pleasure and surrender in each of these feverish stories, and no one walks away from his steamy encounter unsated. Rowberry's men are unafraid to push the limits of civilized behavior in search of the elusive and empowering conquest. One of gay erotica's first success stories.

ROBERT BAHR

SEX SHOW
$4.95/225-6
Luscious dancing boys. Brazen, explicit acts. Unending stimulation. Take a seat, and get very comfortable, because the curtain's going up on a show no discriminating appetite can afford to miss.

JASON FURY

THE ROPE ABOVE, THE BED BELOW
$4.95/269-8
The irresistible Jason Fury returns—this time, telling the tale of a vicious murderer preying upon New York's go-go boy population. No one is who or what they seem, and in order to solve this mystery and save lives, Jason's study suspect must lay bare his soul—and more! Never has a private dick worked so hard!

ERIC'S BODY
$4.95/151-9
Meet Jason Fury—blond, blue-eyed and up for anything. Fury's sexiest tales are collected in book form for the first time. Follow the irresistible Jason through sexual adventures unlike any you have ever read....

MASQUERADE BOOKS

"BIG" BILL JACKSON
EIGHTH WONDER
$4.95/200-0

From the bright lights and back rooms of New York to the open fields and sweaty bods of a small Southern town, "Big" Bill always manages to cause a scene, and the more actors he can involve, the better! Like the man's name says, he's got more than enough for everyone, and turns nobody down....

LARS EIGHNER
WHISPERED IN THE DARK
$5.95/286-2

A volume demonstrating Eighner's unique combination of strengths: poetic descriptive power, an unfailing ear for dialogue, and a finely tuned feeling for the nuances of male passion.

AMERICAN PRELUDE
$4.95/170-5

Eighner is widely recognized as one of our best, most exciting gay writers. He is also one of gay erotica's true masters—and American Prelude shows why. Wonderfully written, blisteringly hot tales of all-American lust.

B.M.O.C.
$4.95/3077-6

In a college town known as "the Athens of the Southwest," studs of every stripe go up all night—studying, naturally. In B.M.O.C., Lars Eighner includes the very best of his short stories, sure to appeal to the collegian in every man. Relive university life the way it was supposed to be, with a cast of handsome honor students majoring in Human Homosexuality.

EDITED BY DAVID LAURENTS
SOUTHERN COMFORT
$6.50/466-6

Editor David Laurents now unleashes another collection of today's most provocative gay writing. The tales here focus on the American South—and reflect not only Southern literary tradition, but the many contributions the region has made to the iconography of the American Male.

WANDERLUST:
HOMOEROTIC TALES OF TRAVEL
$5.95/395-3

A volume dedicated to the special pleasures of faraway places. Gay men have always had a special interest in travel—and not only for the scenic vistas. Wanderlust celebrates the freedom of the open road, and the allure of men who stray from the beaten path....

THE BADBOY BOOK OF EROTIC POETRY
$5.95/382-1

Over fifty of today's best poets. Erotic poetry has long been the problem child of the literary world—highly creative and provocative, but somehow too frank to be "literature." Both learned and stimulating, The Badboy Book of Erotic Poetry restores eros to its rightful place of honor in contemporary gay writing.

AARON TRAVIS
BIG SHOTS
$5.95/448-8

Two electrifying tales in one electrifying volume. In Beirut, Travis tells the story of ultimate military power and erotic subjugation; Kip, Travis' hypersexed and sinister take on film noir, appears in unexpurgated form for the first time—including the final, overwhelming chapter.

EXPOSED
$4.95/126-8

A volume of shorter Travis tales, each providing a unique glimpse of the horny gay male in his natural environment! Cops, college jocks, ancient Romans—even Sherlock Holmes and his loyal Watson—cruise these pages, fresh from the throbbing pen of one of our hottest authors.

BEAST OF BURDEN
$4.95/105-5

Five ferocious tales. Innocents surrender to the brutal sexual mastery of their superiors, as taboos are shattered and replaced with the unwritten rules of masculine conquest. Intense, extreme—and totally Travis.

IN THE BLOOD
$5.95/283-3

Written when Travis had just begun to explore the true power of the erotic imagination, these stories laid the groundwork for later masterpieces. Among the many rewarding rarities included in this volume: "In the Blood" —a heart-pounding descent into sexual vampirism, written with the furious erotic power that has distinguished Travis' work from the beginning.

THE FLESH FABLES
$4.95/243-6

One of Travis' best collections. The Flesh Fables includes "Blue Light," his most famous story, as well as other masterpieces that established him as the erotic writer to watch. And watch carefully, because Travis always buries a surprise somewhere beneath his scorching detail....

SLAVES OF THE EMPIRE
$4.95/3054-7

"Slaves of the Empire is a wonderful mythic tale. Set against the backdrop of the exotic and powerful Roman Empire, this wonderfully written novel explores the timeless questions of light and dark in male sexuality. Travis has shown himself expert in manipulating the most primal themes and images. The locale may be the ancient world, but these are the slaves and masters of our time...."   —John Preston

BOB VICKERY

SKIN DEEP
$4.95/265-5

So many varied beauties no one will go away unsatisfied. No tantalizing morsel of manflesh is overlooked—or left unexplored! Beauty may be only skin deep, but a handful of beautiful skin is a tempting proposition.

JR

FRENCH QUARTER NIGHTS
$5.95/337-6

A randy roundup of this author's most popular tales. *French Quarter Nights* is filled with sensual snapshots of the many places where men get down and dirty—from the steamy French Quarter to the steam room at the old Everard baths. In the best tradition of gay erotica, these are nights you'll wish would go on forever....

TOM BACCHUS

RAHM
$5.95/315-5

The imagination of Tom Bacchus brings to life an extraordinary assortment of characters, from the Father of Us All to the cowpoke next door, the early gay literati to rude, queercore mosh rats. No one is better than Bacchus at staking out sexual territory with a swagger and a sly grin.

BONE
$4.95/177-2

Queer musings from the pen of one of today's hottest young talents. A fresh outlook on fleshly indulgence yields more than a few pleasant surprises. Horny Tom Bacchus maps out the tricking ground of a new generation.

KEY LINCOLN

SUBMISSION HOLDS
$4.95/266-3

A bright young talent unleashes his first collection of gay erotica. From tough to tender, the men between these covers stop at nothing to get what they want. These sweat-soaked tales show just how bad boys can really get—especially when given a little help by an equally lustful stud.

HODDY ALLEN

AL
$5.95/302-3

Al is a remarkable young man. With his long brown hair, bright green eyes and eagerness to please, many would consider him the perfect submissive. Many would like to mark him as their own—but it is at that point that Al stops. One day Al relates the entire astounding tale of his life....

CALDWELL/EIGHNER

QSFX2
$5.95/278-7

The wickedest, wildest, other-worldliest yarns from two master storytellers—Clay Caldwell and Lars Eighner. Both eroticists take a trip to the furthest reaches of the sexual imagination, sending back ten stories proving that as much as things change, one thing will always remain the same....

CLAY CALDWELL

ASK OL' BUDDY
$5.95/346-5

Set in the underground SM world, Caldwell takes you on a journey of discovery—where men initiate one another into the secrets of the rawest sexual realm of all. And when each stud's initiation is complete, he takes his places among the masters—eager to take part in the training of another hungry soul...

STUD SHORTS
$5.95/320-1

"If anything, Caldwell's charm is more powerful, his nostalgia more poignant, the horniness he captures more sweetly, achingly acute than ever."

—Aaron Travis

A new collection of this legend's latest sex-fiction. With his customary candor, Caldwell tells all about cops, cadets, truckers, farmboys (and many more) in these dirty jewels.

TAILPIPE TRUCKER
$5.95/296-5

Trucker porn! In prose as free and unvarnished as a cross-country highway, Caldwell tells the truth about Trag and Curly—two men hot for the feeling of sweaty manflesh. Together, they pick up—and turn out—a couple of thrill-seeking punks.

SERVICE, STUD
$5.95/336-8

Another look at the gay future. The setting is the Los Angeles of a distant future. Here the all-male populace is divided between the served and the servants—guaranteeing the erotic satisfaction of all involved.

QUEERS LIKE US
$4.95/262-0

"This is Caldwell at his most charming."

—Aaron Travis

For years the name Clay Caldwell has been synonymous with the hottest, most finely crafted gay tales available. *Queers Like Us* is one of his best: the story of a randy mailman's trek through a landscape of willing, available studs.

ALL-STUD
$4.95/104-7

This classic, sex-soaked tale takes place under the watchful eye of Number Ten: an omniscient figure who has decreed unabashed promiscuity as the law of his all-male land. One stud, however, takes it upon himself to challenge the social order, daring to fall in love. Finally, he is forced to fight for not only himself, but the man to whom he has committed himself.

CLAY CALDWELL AND AARON TRAVIS

TAG TEAM STUDS
$6.50/465-8

Thrilling tales from these two legendary eroticists. The wrestling world will never seem the same, once you've made your way through this assortment of sweaty, virile studs. But you'd better be wary—should one catch you off guard, you just might spend the rest of the night pinned to the mat.... A double dose of roughstuff, available only from Badboy.

MASQUERADE BOOKS

LARRY TOWNSEND

LEATHER AD: S
$5.95/407-0
The second half of Townsend's acclaimed tale of lust through the personals—this time told from a Top's perspective. A simple ad generates many responses, and one man finds himself in the enviable position of putting these studly applicants through their paces.....

LEATHER AD: M
$5.95/380-5
The first of this two-part classic. John's curious about what goes on between the leatherclad men he's fantasized about. He takes out a personal ad, and starts a journey of self-discovery that will leave no part of his life unchanged.

BEWARE THE GOD WHO SMILES
$5.95/321-X
Two lusty young Americans are transported to ancient Egypt—where they are embroiled in regional warfare and taken as slaves by marauding barbarians. The key to escape from this brutal bondage lies in their own rampant libidos, and urges as old as time itself.

THE CONSTRUCTION WORKER
$5.95/298-1
A young, hung construction worker is sent to a building project in Central America, where he finds that man-to-man sex is the accepted norm. The young stud quickly fits right in—until he senses that beneath the constant sexual shenanigans there moves an almost supernatural force.

2069 TRILOGY
(This one-volume collection only $6.95)244-2
For the first time, Larry Townsend's early science-fiction trilogy appears in one massive volume! Set in a future world, the 2069 Trilogy includes the tight plotting and shameless male sexual pleasure that established him as one of gay erotica's first masters.

MIND MASTER
$4.95/209-4
Who better to explore the territory of erotic dominance than an author who helped define the genre—and knows that ultimate mastery always transcends the physical.

THE LONG LEATHER CORD
$4.95/201-9
Chuck's stepfather never lacks money or clandestine male visitors with whom he enacts intense sexual rituals. As Chuck comes to terms with his own desires, he begins to unravel the mystery behind his stepfather's secret life.

MAN SWORD
$4.95/188-8
France's King Henri III, unimaginably spoiled by his mother—the infamous Catherine de Medici—was groomed from a young age to assume the throne of France. Along the way, he encounters enough sexual schemers and politicos to alter one's picture of history forever!

THE FAUSTUS CONTRACT
$4.95/167-5
Two attractive young men desperately need $1000. Will do anything. Travel OK. Danger OK. Call anytime... Two cocky young hustlers get more than they bargained for in this story of lust and its discontents.

THE GAY ADVENTURES OF CAPTAIN GOOSE
$4.95/169-1
The hot and tender young Jerome Gander is sentenced to serve aboard the H.M.S. Faerigold—a ship manned by the most hardened, unrepentant criminals. In no time, Gander becomes well-versed in the ways of horny men at sea.

CHAINS
$4.95/158-6
Picking up street punks has always been risky, but in Larry Townsend's classic Chains, it sets off a string of events that must be read to be believed.

KISS OF LEATHER
$4.95/161-6
A look at the acts and attitudes of an earlier generation of gay leathermen, Kiss of Leather is full to bursting with the gritty, raw action that has distinguished Townsend's work for years. Pain and pleasure mix in this tightly plotted tale.

RUN, LITTLE LEATHER BOY
$4.95/143-8
One young man's sexual awakening. A chronic underachiever, Wayne seems to be going nowhere fast. He finds himself bored with the everyday—and drawn to the masculine intensity of a dark and mysterious sexual underground....

RUN NO MORE
$4.95/152-7
The continuation of Larry Townsend's legendary Run, Little Leather Boy. This volume follows the further adventures of Townsend's leatherclad narrator as he travels every sexual byway available to the S/M male.

THE SCORPIUS EQUATION
$4.95/119-5
The story of a man caught between the demands of two galactic empires. Our randy hero must match wits—and more—with the incredible forces that rule his world.

THE SEXUAL ADVENTURES OF SHERLOCK HOLMES
$4.95/3097-0
"A Study in Scarlet" is transformed to expose Mrs. Hudson as a man in drag, the Diogenes Club as an S/M arena, and clues only the redoubtable—and very horny—Sherlock Holmes could piece together. A baffling tale of sex and mystery.

MASQUERADE BOOKS

DONALD VINING
CABIN FEVER AND OTHER STORIES
$5.95/338-4

Eighteen blistering stories in celebration of the most intimate of male bonding. Time after time, Donald Vining's men succumb to nature, and reaffirm both love and lust in modern gay life.

"Demonstrates the wisdom experience combined with insight and optimism can create."
—*Bay Area Reporter*

DEREK ADAMS
PRISONER OF DESIRE
$6.50/439-9

Scalding fiction from one of Badboy's most popular authors. The creator of horny P.I. Miles Diamond returns with this volume bursting with red-blooded, sweat-soaked excursions through the modern gay libido.

THE MARK OF THE WOLF
$5.95/361-9

I turned to look at the man who stared back at me from the mirror. The familiar outlines of my face seemed coarser, more sinister. An animal? The past comes back to haunt one well-off stud, whose unslakeable thirsts lead him into the arms of many men—and the midst of a perilous mystery.

MY DOUBLE LIFE
$5.95/314-7

Every man leads a double life, dividing his hours between the mundanities of the day and the outrageous pursuits of the night. The creator of sexy P.I. Miles Diamond shines a little light on the wicked things men do when no one's looking.

BOY TOY
$4.95/260-4

Poor Brendan Callan finds himself the guinea pig of a crazed geneticist. The result: Brendan becomes irresistibly alluring—a talent designed for endless pleasure, but coveted by others for the most unsavory means....

HEAT WAVE
$4.95/159-4

"His body was draped in baggy clothes, but there was hardly any doubt that they covered anything less than perfection.... His slacks were cinched tight around a narrow waist, and the rise of flesh pushing against the thin fabric promised a firm, melon-shaped ass...."

MILES DIAMOND AND THE DEMON OF DEATH
$4.95/251-5

Derek Adams' gay gumshoe returns for further adventures. Miles always find himself in the stickiest situations—with any stud whose path he crosses! His adventures with "The Demon of Death" promise another carnal carnival.

THE ADVENTURES OF MILES DIAMOND
$4.95/118-7

The debut of Miles Diamond—Derek Adams' take on the classic American archetype of the hardboiled private eye. "The Case of the Missing Twin" promises to be a most rewarding case, packed as it is with randy studs. Miles sets about uncovering all as he tracks down the elusive and delectable Daniel Travis. As Miles soon discovers, every man has a secret desire....

KELVIN BELIELE
IF THE SHOE FITS
$4.95/223-X

An essential and winning volume of tales exploring a world where randy boys can't help but do what comes naturally—as often as possible! Sweaty male bodies grapple in pleasure, proving the old adage: if the shoe fits, one might as well slip right in....

VINCE GILMAN
THE SLAVE PRINCE
$4.95/199-3

A runaway royal learns the true meaning of power when he comes under the hand of Korat—a man well-versed in the many ways of subjugating a young man to his relentless sexual appetite.

JAMES MEDLEY
THE REVOLUTIONARY & OTHER STORIES
$6.50/417-8

Billy, the son of the station chief of the American Embassy in Guatemala, is kidnapped and held for ransom. Frightened at first, Billy gradually develops an unimaginably close relationship with Juan, the revolutionary assigned to guard him. Things soon heat up—thanks to Medley's unforgettable mixture of high adventure and unquenchable lust!

HUCK AND BILLY
$4.95/245-0

Young love is always the sweetest, always the most sorrowful. Young lust, on the other hand, knows no bounds—and is often the hottest of one's life! Huck and Billy explore the desires that course through their young male bodies, determined to plumb the lusty depths of passion.

FLEDERMAUS
FLEDERFICTION:
STORIES OF MEN AND TORTURE
$5.95/355-4

Fifteen blistering paeans to men and their suffering. Fledermaus unleashes his most thrilling tales of punishment in this special volume designed with Badboy readers in mind.

VICTOR TERRY
MASTERS
$6.50/418-6

A powerhouse volume of boot-wearing, whip-wielding, bone-crunching bruisers who've got what it takes to make a grown man grovel. From a chance encounter on the Christopher Street pier to an impromptu session with a mysterious and unrelenting visitor, this collection focuses on the most demanding of men—the imperious few to whom so many humbly offer themselves....

SM/SD
$6.50/406-2

Set around a South Dakota town called Prairie, these tales offer compelling evidence that the real rough stuff can still be found where men roam free of the restraints of "polite" society—and take what they want despite all rules.

MASQUERADE BOOKS

CARO SOLES & STAN TAL, EDITORS
BIZARRE DREAMS
$4.95/187-2
An anthology of stirring voices dedicated to exploring the dark side of human fantasy. *Bizarre Dreams* brings together the most talented practitioners of "dark fantasy," the most forbidden sexual realm of all.

CHRISTOPHER MORGAN
STEAM GAUGE
$6.50/473-9
The first collection of short stories from the author of the bestselling *Muscle Bound*. This volume abounds in manly men doing what they do best—to, with, or for any hot stud who crosses their paths. Frequently published to acclaim in the gay press, Christopher Morgan puts a fresh, contemporary spin on the very oldest of urges.
THE SPORTSMEN
$5.95/385-6
A collection of super-hot stories dedicated to that most popular of boys next door—the all-American athlete. Here are enough tales of carnal grand slams, sexy interceptions and highly personal bests to satisfy the hungers of the most ardent sports fan. Editor Christopher Morgan has gathered those writers who know just the type of guys that make up every red-blooded male's starting line-up....
MUSCLE BOUND
$4.95/3028-8
In the New York City bodybuilding scene, country boy Tommy joins forces with sexy Will Rodriguez in a battle of wits and biceps at the hottest gym in town, where the weak are bound and crushed by iron-pumping gods.

DAVE KINNICK
SORRY I ASKED
$4.95/3090-3
Unexpurgated interviews with gay porn's rank and file. Get personal with the men behind (and under) the "stars," and discover the hot truth about the porn business.

MICHAEL LOWENTHAL, ED.
THE BADBOY EROTIC LIBRARY VOLUME I
$4.95/190-X
Excerpts from *A Secret Life, Imre, Sins of the Cities of the Plain, Teleny* and others demonstrate the uncanny gift for portraying sex between men that led to many of these titles being banned upon publication.
THE BADBOY EROTIC LIBRARY VOLUME II
$4.95/211-6
This time, selections are taken from *Mike and Me* and *Muscle Bound, Men at Work, Badboy Fantasies,* and *Slowburn.*

ERIC BOYD
MIKE AND ME
$5.95/419-4
Mike joined the gym squad to bulk up on muscle. Little did he know he'd be turning on every sexy muscle jock in Minnesota! Hard bodies collide in a series of workouts designed to generate a whole lot more than rips and cuts.

MIKE AND THE MARINES
$6.50/497-6
Mike takes on America's most elite corps of studs—running into more than a few good men! Join in on the never-ending sexual escapades of this singularly lustful platoon!

ANONYMOUS
A SECRET LIFE
$4.95/3017-2
Meet Master Charles: only eighteen, and quite innocent, until his arrival at the Sir Percival's Royal Academy, where the daily lessons are supplemented with a crash course in pure, sweet sexual heat!
SINS OF THE CITIES OF THE PLAIN
$5.95/322-8
ndulge yourself in the scorching memoirs of young man-about-town Jack Saul. With his shocking dalliances with the lords and "ladies" of British high society, Jack's positively sinful escapades grow wilder with every chapter!
IMRE
$4.95/3019-9
What dark secrets, what fiery passions lay hidden behind strikingly beautiful Lieutenant Imre's emerald eyes? An extraordinary lost classic of fantasy, obsession, gay erotic desire, and romance in a small European town on the eve of WWI.
TELENY
$4.95/3020-2
Often attributed to Oscar Wilde, *Teleny* tells the story of one young man of independent means. He dedicates himself to a succession of forbidden pleasures, but instead finds love and tragedy when he becomes embroiled in a cult devoted to fulfilling only the very darkest of fantasies.

PAT CALIFIA
THE SEXPERT
$4.95/3034-2
You can turn to for one authority for answers to virtually any question on the subjects of intimacy and sexual performance—The Sexpert, who responds to real-life sexual concerns with uncanny wisdom and a razor wit.

HARD CANDY

PATRICK MOORE
IOWA
$6.95/423-2
"Moore is the Tennessee Williams of the nineties—profound intimacy freed in a compelling narrative."
—Karen Finley
"Fresh and shiny and relevant to our time. *Iowa* is full of terrific characters etched in acid-sharp prose, soaked through with just enough ambivalence to make it thoroughly romantic."
—Felice Picano
A stunning novel about one gay man's journey into adulthood, and the roads that bring him home again. From the author of the highly praised *This Every Night.*

MASQUERADE BOOKS

STAN LEVENTHAL

BARBIE IN BONDAGE
$6.95/415-1

Widely regarded as one of the most refreshing, clear-eyed interpreters of big city gay male life, Leventhal here provides a series of explorations of love and desire between men. Uncompromising, but gentle and generous, *Barbie in Bondage* is a fitting tribute to the late author's unique talents.

SKYDIVING ON CHRISTOPHER STREET
$6.95/287-6

"Positively addictive."   —Dennis Cooper

Aside from a hateful job, a hateful apartment, a hateful world and an increasingly hateful lover, life seems, well, all right for the protagonist of Stan Leventhal's latest novel. Having already lost most of his friends to AIDS, how could things get any worse? But things soon do, and he's forced to endure much more....

PAUL T. ROGERS

SAUL'S BOOK
$7.95/462-3

Winner of the First Annual Editors' Book Award

"Exudes an almost narcotic power.... A masterpiece."
                    —*Village Voice Literary Supplement*

"A first novel of considerable power... Sinbad the Sailor, thanks to the sympathetic imagination of Paul T. Rogers, speaks to us all."   —*New York Times Book Review*

The story of a Times Square hustler called Sinbad the Sailor and Saul, a brilliant, self-destructive, alcoholic, thoroughly dominating character who may be the only love Sindab will ever know.

WALTER HOLLAND

THE MARCH
$6.95/429-1

A moving testament to the power of friendship during even the worst of times. Beginning on a hot summer night in 1980, *The March* revolves around a circle of young gay men, and the many others their lives touch. Over time, each character changes in unexpected ways; lives and loves come together and fall apart, as society itself is horribly altered by the onslaught of AIDS. A kaleidoscopic portrait of friendship, love, loss, and the myriad triumphs and devastations of contemporary life. From the acclaimed author of *A Journal of the Plague Years*.

RED JORDAN AROBATEAU

LUCY AND MICKEY
$6.95/311-2

The story of Mickey—an uncompromising butch—and her long affair with Lucy, the femme she loves.A raw tale of pre-Stonewall lesbian life.

"A necessary reminder to all who blissfully—some may say ignorantly—ride the wave of lesbian chic into the mainstream."   —Heather Findlay

DIRTY PICTURES
$5.95/345-7

"Red Jordan Arobateau is the Thomas Wolfe of lesbian literature... Arobateau's work overflows with vitality and pulsing life. She's a natural—raw talent that is seething, passionate, hard, remarkable."
        —Lillian Faderman, editor of *Chloe Plus Olivia*

Dirty Pictures is the story of a lonely butch tending bar—and the femme she finally calls her own.

DONALD VINING

A GAY DIARY
$8.95/451-8

Donald Vining's *Diary* portrays a long-vanished age and the lifestyle of a gay generation all too frequently forgotten. A touching and revealing volume documenting the surprisingly vibrant culture that existed decades before Stonewall.

"*A Gay Diary* is, unquestionably, the richest historical document of gay male life in the United States that I have ever encountered.... It illuminates a critical period in gay male American history."
        —*Body Politic*

LARS EIGHNER

GAY COSMOS
$6.95/236-1

A title sure to appeal not only to Eighner's gay fans, but the many converts who first encountered his moving nonfiction work. Praised by the press, *Gay Cosmos* is an important contribution to the burgeoning area of Gay and Lesbian Studies—and sure to provoke many readers.

FELICE PICANO

THE LURE
$6.95/398-8

"The subject matter, plus the authenticity of Picano's research are, combined, explosive. Felice Picano is one hell of a writer."   —Stephen King

After witnessing a brutal murder, Noel is recruited by the police, to assist as a lure for the killer. Undercover, he moves deep into the freneticism of Manhattan's gay highlife—where he gradually becomes aware of the darker forces at work in his life. In addition to the mystery behind his mission, he begins to recognize changes: in his relationships with the men around him, in himself...

AMBIDEXTROUS
$6.95/275-2

"Deftly evokes those placid Eisenhower years of bicycles, boners, and book reports. Makes us remember what it feels like to be a child..."
        —*The Advocate*

Picano's first "memoir in the form of a novel" tells all: home life, school face-offs, the ingenuous sophistications of his first sexual steps. In three years' time, he's had his first gay fling—and is on his way to becoming the widely praised writer he is today.

MASQUERADE BOOKS

MEN WHO LOVED ME
$6.95/274-4

"Zesty...spiked with adventure and romance...a distinguished and humorous portrait of a vanished age."
—Publishers Weekly

In 1966, Picano abandoned New York, determined to find true love in Europe. When the older and wiser Picano returns to New York at last, he plunges into the city's thriving gay community—experiencing the frenzy and heartbreak that came to define Greenwich Village society in the 1970s.

WILLIAM TALSMAN
THE GAUDY IMAGE
$6.95/263-9

"To read *The Gaudy Image* now...it is to see first-hand the very issues of identity and positionality with which gay men were struggling in the decades before Stonewall. For what Talsman is dealing with...is the very question of how we conceive ourselves gay."
—from the introduction by Michael Bronski

ROSEBUD

THE ROSEBUD READER
$5.95/319-8

Rosebud has contributed greatly to the burgeoning genre of lesbian erotica—to the point that authors like Lindsay Welsh, Aarona Griffin and Valentina Cilescu are among the hottest and most closely watched names in lesbian and gay publishing. Here are the finest moments from Rosebud's contemporary classics.

RANDY TUROFF
LUST NEVER SLEEPS
$6.50/475-5

A powerful volume of highly erotic, touchingly real fiction from the editor of *Lesbian Words*. Turoff accurately and insightfully depicts a circle of modern women, telling the stories of their lives and loves through a series of interconnected stories. Like the stories in *Lust Never Sleeps*, each of Turoff's women very capably stands on her own two feet—even while gaining resonance and deeper meaning from the relationships she has built to the others in her world. A stirring evocation of contemporary lesbian community.

RED JORDAN AROBATEAU
ROUGH TRADE
$6.50/470-4

Famous for her unflinching portrayal of lower-class dyke life and love, Arobateau outdoes herself with these tales of butch/femme affairs and unrelenting passions. Unapologetic and distinctly non-homogenized, *Rough Trade* is a must for all fans of challenging lesbian literature.

BOYS NIGHT OUT
$6.50/463-1

A *Red*-hot volume of short fiction from this lesbian literary sensation. As always, Arobateau takes a good hard look at the lives of everyday women, noting well the struggles and triumphs each woman experiences. Never one to shrink from the less-than-chic truth, Red Jordan Arobateau has carved herself a niche as the foremost chronicler of working class dyke life.

ALISON TYLER
DARK ROOM: AN ONLINE ADVENTURE
$6.50/455-0

Dani, a successful photographer, can't bring herself to face the death of her lover, Kate. An ambitious journalist, Kate was found mysteriously murdered, leaving her lover with only fond memories of a too-brief relationship. Determined to keep the memory of her lover alive, Dani goes online under Kate's screen alias—and begins to uncover the truth behind the crime that has torn her world apart.

BLUE SKY SIDEWAYS & OTHER STORIES
$6.50/394-5

A variety of women, and their many breathtaking experiences with lovers, friends—and even the occasional sexy stranger. From blossoming young beauties to fearless vixens, Tyler finds the sexy pleasures of everyday life.

DIAL "L" FOR LOVELESS
$5.95/386-4

Meet Katrina Loveless—a private eye talented enough to give Sam Spade a run for his money. In her first case, Katrina investigates a murder implicating a host of society's darlings—including wealthy Tessa and Baxter Saint Claire, and the lovely, tantalizing, infamous Geneva twins. Loveless untangles the mess— while working herself into a variety of highly compromising knots with the many lovelies who cross her path!

THE VIRGIN
$5.95/379-1

Veronica answers a personal ad in the "Women Seeking Women" category—and discovers a whole sensual world she never knew existed! And she never dreamed she'd be prized as a virgin all over again, by someone who would deflower her with a passion no man could ever show....

THE BLUE ROSE
$5.95/335-X

The tale of a modern sorority—fashioned after a Victorian girls' school. Ignited to the heights of passion by erotic tales of the Victorian age, a group of lusty young women are encouraged to act out their forbidden fantasies—all under the tutelage of Mistresses Emily and Justine, two avid practitioners of hard-core discipline!

K. T. BUTLER
TOOLS OF THE TRADE
$5.95/420-8

A sparkling mix of lesbian erotica and humor. An encounter with ice cream, cappuccino and chocolate cake; an affair with a complete stranger; a pair of faulty handcuffs; and love on a drafting table. Seventeen tales.

MASQUERADE BOOKS

LOVECHILD

GAG
$5.95/369-4

From New York's poetry scene comes this explosive volume of work from one of the bravest, most cutting young writers you'll ever encounter. The poems in *Gag* take on American hypocrisy with uncommon energy, and announce Lovechild as a writer of unforgettable rage.

ELIZABETH OLIVER

THE SM MURDER: MURDER AT ROMAN HILL
$5.95/353-8

Intrepid lesbian P.I.s Leslie Patrick and Robin Penny take on a really hot case: the murder of the notorious Felicia Roman. The circumstances of the crime lead the pair on an excursion through the leatherdyke underground, where motives—and desires—run deep.

PAGAN DREAMS
$5.95/295-7

Cassidy and Samantha plan a vacation at a secluded bed-and-breakfast, hoping for a little personal time alone. Their hostess, however, has different plans. The lovers are plunged into a world of dungeons and pagan rites, as Anastasia steals Samantha for her own.

SUSAN ANDERS

CITY OF WOMEN
$5.95/375-9

Stories dedicated to women and the passions that draw them together. Designed strictly for the sensual pleasure of women, these tales are set to ignite flames of passion from coast to coast.

PINK CHAMPAGNE
$5.95/282-5

Tasty, torrid tales of butch/femme couplings. Tough as nails or soft as silk, these women seek out their antitheses, intent on working out the details of their own personal theory of difference.

ANONYMOUS

LAVENDER ROSE
$4.95/208-6

From the writings of Sappho, Queen of the island Lesbos, to the turn-of-the-century *Black Book of Lesbianism*; from *Tips to Maidens* to *Crimson Hairs*, a recent lesbian saga—here are the great but little-known lesbian writings and revelations. A one volume survey of hot and historic lesbian writing.

LAURA ANTONIOU, EDITOR

LEATHERWOMEN
$4.95/3095-1

These fantasies, from the pens of new or emerging authors, break every rule imposed on women's fantasies. The hottest stories from some of today's newest and most outrageous writers make this an unforgettable exploration of the female libido.

LEATHERWOMEN II
$4.95/229-9

Writings of women on the edge—resulting in a collection sure to ignite libidinal flames. Leave taboos behind, because these Leatherwomen know no limits....

AARONA GRIFFIN

PASSAGE AND OTHER STORIES
$4.95/3057-1

An S/M romance. Lovely Nina is frightened by her lesbian passions, until she finds herself infatuated with a woman she spots at a local café. One night Nina follows her, and finds herself enmeshed in an endless maze leading to a world where women test the edges of sexuality and power.

VALENTINA CILESCU

MY LADY'S PLEASURE:
WOMAN WITH A MAID VOLUME I
$5.95/412-7

Dr. Claudia Dungarrow, a lovely, powerful, but mysterious figure at St. Matilda's College, attempts to seduce virginal Elizabeth Stanbridge, she sets off a chain of events that eventually ruins her career. Claudia vows revenge—and makes her foes pay deliciously....

DARK VENUS:
MISTRESS WITH A MAID, VOLUME 2
$6.50/481-X

This thrilling saga of cruel lust continues! *Mistress with a Maid* breathes new life into the conventions of dominance and submission. What emerges is a picture of unremitting desire—whether it be for supreme erotic power or ultimate sexual surrender.

THE ROSEBUD SUTRA
$4.95/242-6

"Women are hardly ever known in their true light, though they may love others, or become indifferent towards them, may give them delight, or abandon them, or may extract from them all the wealth that they possess." So says *The Rosebud Sutra*—a volume promising women's inner secrets. One woman learns to use these secrets in a quest for pleasure with a succession of lady loves....

THE HAVEN
$4.95/165-9

J craves domination, and her perverse appetites lead her to the Haven: the isolated sanctuary Ros and Annie call home. Soon J forces her way into the couple's world, bringing unspeakable lust and cruelty into their lives.

MISTRESS MINE
$5.95/445-3

Sophia Cranleigh sits in prison, accused of authoring the "obscene" *Mistress Mine*. What she has done, however, is merely chronicle the events of her life—to the outrage of many. For Sophia has led no ordinary life, but has slaved and suffered—deliciously—under the hand of the notorious Mistress Malin. How long had she languished under the dominance of this incredible beauty?

MASQUERADE BOOKS

LINDSAY WELSH

SECOND SIGHT
$6.50/507-7

The debut of Dana Steele—lesbian superhero!
During an attack by a gang of homophobic youths, Dana is thrown onto subway tracks—touching the deadly third rail. Miraculously, she survives, and finds herself endowed with superhuman powers. Not wishing to waste her extraordinary new lease on life, Dana decides to devote her powers to the protection of her lesbian sisters, no matter how daunting the danger they face. With the help of her lover Astrid, Dana stands poised to become a legend in her own time.

NASTY PERSUASIONS
$6.50/436-4

A hot peek into the behind-the-scenes operations of Rough Trade—one of the world's most famous lesbian clubs. Join Slash, Ramone, Cherry and many others as they bring one another to the height of torturous ecstasy—all in the name of keeping Rough Trade the premier name in sexy entertainment for women.

MILITARY SECRETS
$5.95/397-X

Colonel Candice Sproule heads a highly specialized boot camp. Assisted by three dominatrix sergeants, Col. Sproule takes on the talented submissives sent to her by secret military contacts. Then comes Jesse—whose pleasure in being served matches the Colonel's own. This new recruit sets off fireworks in the barracks—and beyond....

ROMANTIC ENCOUNTERS
$5.95/359-7

Beautiful Julie, the most powerful editor of romance novels in the industry, spends her days igniting women's passions through books—and her nights fulfilling those needs with a variety of lovers. Finally, through a sizzling series of coincidences, Julie's two worlds come together explosively!

THE BEST OF LINDSAY WELSH
$5.95/368-6

A collection of this popular writer's best work. This author was one of Rosebud's early bestsellers, and remains highly popular. A sampler set to introduce some of the hottest lesbian erotica to a wider audience.

NECESSARY EVIL
$5.95/277-9

What's a girl to do? When her Mistress proves too systematic, too by-the-book, one lovely submissive takes the ultimate chance—choosing and creating a Mistress who'll fulfill her heart's desire. Little did she know how difficult it would be—and, in the end, rewarding....

A VICTORIAN ROMANCE
$5.95/365-1

Lust-letters from the road. A young Englishwoman realizes her dream—a trip abroad under the guidance of her eccentric maiden aunt. Soon, the young but blossoming Elaine comes to discover her own sexual talents, as a hot-blooded Parisian named Madelaine takes her Sapphic education in hand.

A CIRCLE OF FRIENDS
$4.95/250-7

The story of a remarkable group of women. The women pair off to explore all the possibilities of lesbian passion, until finally it seems that there is nothing—and no one—they have not dabbled in.

BAD HABITS
$5.95/446-1

What does one do with a poorly trained slave? Break her of her bad habits, of course! The story of the ultimate finishing school, *Bad Habits* was an immediate favorite with women nationwide.

"Talk about passing the wet test!... If you like hot, lesbian erotica, run—don't walk—and pick up a copy of *Bad Habits*." —*Lambda Book Repor*

ANNABELLE BARKER

MOROCCO
$4.95/148-9

A luscious young woman stands to inherit a fortune—if she can only withstand the ministrations of her cruel guardian until her twentieth birthday. With two months left, Lila makes a bold bid for freedom, only to find that liberty has its own excruciating and delicious price....

A.L. REINE

DISTANT LOVE & OTHER STORIES
$4.95/3056-3

In the title story, Leah Michaels and her lover, Ranelle, have had four years of blissful, smoldering passion together. When Ranelle is out of town, Leah records an audio "Valentine:" a cassette filled with erotic reminiscences....

A RICHARD KASAK BOOK

EDITED BY SHAR REDNOUR

VIRGIN TERRITORY 2
$12.95/506-9

The follow-up volume to the groundbreaking *Virgin Territory*. This volume includes the work of many woman inspired by the success of *VT*, and their stories should prove just as liberating. Focusing on the many "firsts" of a woman's erotic life, *Virgin Territory 2* provides one of the sole outlets for serious discussion of the myriad possibilities available to and chosen by many contemporary lesbians. A necessary addition to the library of any reader interested in the state of contemporary sexuality.

VIRGIN TERRITORY
$12.95/457-7

An anthology of writing by women about their first-time erotic experiences with other women. From the longings and ecstasies of awakening dykes to the sometimes awkward pleasures of sexual experimentation on the edge, each of these true stories reveals a different, radical perspective on one of the most traditional subjects around: virginity.

MASQUERADE BOOKS

MICHAEL FORD, EDITOR
ONCE UPON A TIME:
EROTIC FAIRY TALES FOR WOMEN
$12.95/449-6

How relevant to contemporary lesbians are the lessons of these age-old tales? The contributors to *Once Upon a Time*—some of the biggest names in contemporary lesbian literature—retell their favorite fairy tales, adding their own surprising—and sexy—twists. *Once Upon a Time* is sure to be one of contemporary lesbian literature's classic collections.

HAPPILY EVER AFTER:
EROTIC FAIRY TALES FOR MEN
$12.95/450-X

A hefty volume of bedtime stories Mother Goose never thought to write down. Adapting some of childhood's most beloved tales for the adult gay reader, the contributors to *Happily Ever After* dig the subtext of these hitherto "innocent" diversions—adding some surprises of their own along the way.

MICHAEL BRONSKI, EDITOR
TAKING LIBERTIES: GAY MEN'S ESSAYS
ON POLITICS, CULTURE AND SEX
$12.95/456-9

"Offers undeniable proof of a heady, sophisticated, diverse new culture of gay intellectual debate. I cannot recommend it too highly."—Christopher Bram

A collection of some of the most divergent views on the state of contemporary gay male culture published in recent years. Michael Bronski here presents some of the community's foremost essayists weighing in on such slippery topics as outing, masculine identity, pornography, the pedophile movement, political strategy—and much more. Includes essays by Pulitzer Prize-winning playwright Tony Kushner, conservative firebrands Bruce Bawer and Andrew Sullivan, literary sensation John Preston, and many others.

FLASHPOINT: GAY MALE SEXUAL WRITING
$12.95/424-0

A collection of the most provocative testaments to gay eros. Michael Bronski presents over twenty of the genre's best writers, exploring areas such as Enlightenment, True Life Adventures and more. Sure to be one of the most talked about and influential volumes ever dedicated to the exploration of gay sexuality.

HEATHER FINDLAY, EDITOR
A MOVEMENT OF EROS:
25 YEARS OF LESBIAN EROTICA
$12.95/421-6

One of the most scintillating overviews of lesbian erotic writing ever published. Heather Findlay has assembled a roster of stellar talents, each represented by their best work. Tracing the course of the genre from its pre-Stonewall roots to its current renaissance, Findlay examines each piece, placing it within the context of lesbian community and politics.

CHARLES HENRI FORD & PARKER TYLER
THE YOUNG AND EVIL
$12.95/431-3

"*The Young and Evil* creates [its] generation as *This Side of Paradise* by Fitzgerald created his generation."
—Gertrude Stein

Originally published in 1933, *The Young and Evil* was an immediate sensation due to its unprecedented portrayal of young gay artists living in New York's notorious Greenwich Village. From flamboyant drag balls to squalid bohemian flats, these characters followed love and art wherever it led them—with a frankness that had the novel banned for many years.

MICHAEL ROWE
WRITING BELOW THE BELT:
CONVERSATIONS WITH EROTIC AUTHORS
$19.95/363-5

"An in-depth and enlightening tour of society's love/hate relationship with sex, morality, and censorship."
—James White Review

Journalist Michael Rowe interviewed the best erotic writers and presents the collected wisdom in *Writing Below the Belt*. Rowe speaks frankly with cult favorites such as Pat Califia, crossover success stories like John Preston, and up-and-comers Michael Lowenthal and Will Leber. A volume dedicated to chronicling the insights of some of this overlooked genre's most renowned practitioners. An acclaimed look at this vital literature.

LARRY TOWNSEND
ASK LARRY
$12.95/289-2

One of the leather community's most respected scribes here presents the best of his advice to leathermen worldwide. Starting just before the onslaught of AIDS, Townsend wrote the "Leather Notebook" column for *Drummer* magazine. Now, readers can avail themselves of Townsend's collected wisdom, as well as the author's contemporary commentary—a careful consideration of the way life has changed in the AIDS era. From Daddies to dog collars, and belts to bruises, *Ask Larry* is an essential volume for any man worth his leathers.

MICHAEL LASSELL
THE HARD WAY
$12.95/231-0

"Lassell is a master of the necessary word. In an age of tepid and whining verse, his bawdy and bittersweet songs are like a plunge in cold champagne."
—Paul Monette

The first collection of renowned gay writer Michael Lassell's poetry, fiction and essays. As much a chronicle of post-Stonewall gay life as a compendium of a remarkable writer's work.

MASQUERADE BOOKS

AMARANTHA KNIGHT, EDITOR
OVE BITES
$12.95/234-5

volume of tales dedicated to legend's sexiest demon—
he Vampire. Not only the finest collection of erotic horror
vailable—but a virtual who's who of promising new
alent. A must for fans of both the horror and erotic genres.

RANDY TUROFF, EDITOR
ESBIAN WORDS: STATE OF THE ART
$10.95/340-6

"This is a terrific book that should be on every think-
ng lesbian's bookshelf."
—Nisa Donnelly
One of the widest assortments of lesbian nonfiction writing
n one revealing volume. Dorothy Allison, Jewelle Gomez,
udy Grahn, Eileen Myles, Robin Podolsky and many others
re represented by some of their best work, looking at not
nly the current fashionability the media has brought to the
esbian "image," but important considerations of the
esbian past via historical inquiry and personal recollec-
ions.

ASSOTTO SAINT
SPELLS OF A VOODOO DOLL
$12.95/393-7

"Angelic and brazen."—Jewelle Gomez
A fierce, spellbinding collection of the poetry, lyrics, essays
and performance texts of Assotto Saint—one of the most
mportant voices in the renaissance of black gay writing.
Saint, aka Yves François Lubin, was the editor of two semi-
nal anthologies: 1991 Lambda Literary Book Award
winner, *The Road Before Us: 100 Gay Black Poets* and
Here to Dare: 10 Gay Black Poets. He was also the author
of two books of poetry, *Stations* and *Wishing for Wings*.

WILLIAM CARNEY
THE REAL THING
$10.95/280-9

"Carney gives us a good look at the mores and
ifestyle of the first generation of gay leathermen. A
chilling mystery/romance novel as well."—Pat Califia
With a new introduction by Michael Bronski. *The Real
Thing* has long served as a touchstone in any consideration
of gay "edge fiction." First published in 1968, this uncompromising story of American leathermen received instant
acclaim. *The Real Thing* finally returns from exile, ready to
thrill a new generation.

EURYDICE
F/32
$10.95/350-3

"It's wonderful to see a woman...celebrating her
body and her sexuality by creating a fabulous and
funny tale."
—Kathy Acker
With the story of Ela, Eurydice won the National Fiction
competition sponsored by Fiction Collective Two and Illinois
State University. A funny, disturbing quest for unity, *f/32*
prompted Frederic Tuten to proclaim "almost any page...
redeems us from the anemic writing and banalities we
have endured in the past decade..."

SAMUEL R. DELANY
THE MOTION OF LIGHT IN WATER
$12.95/133-0

"A very moving, intensely fascinating literary biog-
raphy from an extraordinary writer. Thoroughly
admirable candor and luminous stylistic precision;
the artist as a young man and a memorable picture
of an age."
—William Gibson
Award-winning author Samuel R. Delany's autobiography
covers the early years of one of science fiction's most
important voices. *The Motion of Light in Water* follows
Delany from his early marriage to the poet Marilyn Hacker,
through the publication of his first, groundbreaking work.
Delany paints a vivid and compelling picture of New York's
East Village in the early '60s.

THE MAD MAN
$23.95/193-4/hardcover

Delany's fascinating examination of human desire. For his
thesis, graduate student John Marr researches the life and
work of the brilliant Timothy Hasler: a philosopher whose
career was cut tragically short over a decade earlier. Marr
soon begins to believe that Hasler's death might hold some
key to his own life as a gay man in the age of AIDS.
"What Delany has done here is take the ideas of the
Marquis de Sade one step further, by filtering
extreme and obsessive sexual behavior through the
sieve of post-modern experience...."
—Lambda Book Report
"Delany develops an insightful dichotomy between
[his protagonist]'s two worlds: the one of cerebral
philosophy and dry academia, the other of heedless,
'impersonal' obsessive sexual extremism. When
these worlds finally collide ... the novel achieves a
surprisingly satisfying resolution...."
—Publishers Weekly

BARRY HOFFMAN, EDITOR
THE BEST OF GAUNTLET
$12.95/202-7

Gauntlet has, with its semi-annual issues, always publishing the widest possible range of opinions. The most
provocative articles have been gathered by editor-in-chief
Barry Hoffman, to make *The Best of Gauntlet* a riveting
exploration of American society's limits.

FELICE PICANO
DRYLAND'S END
$12.95/279-5

The science fiction debut of the highly acclaimed author of
Men Who Loved Me and *Like People in History*. Set five
thousand years in the future, *Dryland's End* takes place in a
fabulous techno-empire ruled by intelligent, powerful
women. While the Matriarchy has ruled for over two thousand years and altered human language, thought and
society, it is now unraveling. Military rivalries, religious
fanaticism and economic competition threaten to destroy
the mighty empire. A Lambda Literary Award nominee in
the Science Fiction category, Picano's first foray into the
genre has met with a wildly enthusiastic response.

MASQUERADE BOOKS

ROBERT PATRICK
TEMPLE SLAVE
$12.95/191-8

"You must read this book." —Quentin Crisp

"This is nothing less than the secret history of the most theatrical of theaters, the most bohemian of Americans and the most knowing of queens. Patrick writes with a lush and witty abandon, as if this departure from the crafting of plays has energized him. *Temple Slave* is also one of the best ways to learn what it was like to be fabulous, gay, theatrical and loved in a time at once more and less dangerous to gay life than our own." —*Genre*

The fascinating, fictionalized tale of the birth of gay theater, from this award-winning playwright.

CHEA VILLANUEVA
JESSIE'S SONG
$9.95/235-3

"It conjures up the strobe-light confusion and excitement of urban dyke life.... Read about these dykes and you'll love them." —Rebecca Ripley

Based largely upon her own experience, Villanueva's work is remarkable for its frankness, and delightful in its iconoclasm. Unconcerned with political correctness, this writer has helped expand the boundaries of "serious" lesbian writing.

GUILLERMO BOSCH
RAIN
$12.95/232-9

"Rain is a trip..." —Timothy Leary

An adult fairy tale, *Rain* takes place in a time when the mysteries of Eros are played out against a background of uncommon deprivation. The tale begins on the 1,537th day of drought—when one man comes to know the true depths of thirst. In a quest to sate his hunger for some knowledge of the wide world, he is taken through a series of extraordinary, unearthly encounters that promise to change not only his life, but the course of civilization around him. A haunting and provocative debut, and a moving fable for our time.

LAURA ANTONIOU, EDITOR
LOOKING FOR MR. PRESTON
$23.95/288-4

Edited by Laura Antoniou, *Looking for Mr. Preston* includes work by Lars Eighner, Pat Califia, Michael Bronski, Joan Nestle, and others who contributed interviews, essays and personal reminiscences of John Preston—a man whose career spanned the industry. Preston was the author of over twenty books, and edited many more. Ten percent of the proceeds from sale of the book will go to the AIDS Project of Southern Maine, for which Preston served as President of the Board.

CECILIA TAN, EDITOR
SM VISIONS: THE BEST OF CIRCLET PRESS
$10.95/339-2

"Fabulous books! There's nothing else like them."
—Susie Bright,
Best American Erotica and Herotica 3

Circlet Press, devoted exclusively to the erotic science fiction and fantasy genre, is now represented by the best of its very best: *SM Visions*—sure to be one of the most thrilling and eye-opening rides through the erotic imagination ever published.

KATHLEEN K.
SWEET TALKERS
$12.95/192-6

Kathleen K., a highly successful businesswoman, opens up her diary for a rare peek at her day-to-day life. What makes Kathleen's story unusual is the nature of her business—she is a popular phone sex operator, and she now reveals a number of secrets and surprises.

RUSS KICK
OUTPOSTS:
A CATALOG OF RARE AND DISTURBING ALTERNATIVE INFORMATION
$18.95/0202-8

A huge, authoritative guide to some of the most bizarre publications available today! Rather than simply summarize the plethora of opinions crowding the American scene, Kick has tracked down and compiled reviews of work penned by political extremists, conspiracy theorists, hallucinogenic pathfinders, sexual explorers, and others. Each review is followed by ordering information for the many readers sure to want these publications for themselves.

MICHAEL LOWENTHAL, EDITOR
THE BEST OF THE BADBOYS
$12.95/233-7

The very best of the leading Badboys is collected here, in this testament to the artistry that has catapulted these "outlaw" authors to bestselling status. John Preston, Aaron Travis, Larry Townsend, and others are here represented by their most provocative writing.

LUCY TAYLOR
UNNATURAL ACTS
$12.95/181-0

"A topnotch collection..." —*Science Fiction Chronicle*

Unnatural Acts plunges deep into the dark side of the psyche and brings to life a disturbing vision of erotic horror. Unrelenting angels and hungry gods play with souls and bodies in Taylor's murky cosmos: where heaven and hell are merely differences of perspective; where redemption and damnation lie behind the same shocking acts. A frightening look at the disturbing, dark side of human desire, and the uncharted territory between life and death.

MASQUERADE BOOKS

TIM WOODWARD, EDITOR
THE BEST OF SKIN TWO
$12.95/130-6

A groundbreaking journal from the crossroads of sexuality, fashion, and art, *Skin Two* specializes in provocative essays by the finest writers working in the "radical sex" scene. Collected here are the articles and interviews that established the magazine's reputation. Including interviews with cult figures Tim Burton, Clive Barker and Jean Paul Gaultier.

MICHAEL PERKINS
THE GOOD PARTS: AN UNCENSORED GUIDE TO LITERARY SEXUALITY
$12.95/186-1

Michael Perkins, one of America's only critics to regularly scrutinize sexual literature, presents sex as seen in the pages of over 100 major fiction and nonfiction volumes from the past twenty years. A one-of-a-kind compendium of "mainstream" sex-writing.
COMING UP:
THE WORLD'S BEST EROTIC WRITING
$12.95/370-8

Author and critic Michael Perkins has scoured the field of erotic writing to produce this anthology sure to challenge the limits of even the most seasoned reader. Using the same sharp eye and transgressive instinct that have established him as America's leading commentator on sexually explicit fiction, Perkins here presents the cream of the current crop.

DAVID MELTZER
THE AGENCY TRILOGY
$12.95/216-7

"... The Agency' is clearly Meltzer's paradigm of society; a mindless machine of which we are all 'agents,' including those whom the machine supposedly serves...."
—Norman Spinrad

When first published, *The Agency* explored issues of erotic dominance and submission with an immediacy and frankness previously unheard of in American literature, as well as presented a vision of an America consumed and dehumanized by a lust for power.

JOHN PRESTON
MY LIFE AS A PORNOGRAPHER AND OTHER INDECENT ACTS
$12.95/135-7

"...essential and enlightening... [My Life as a Pornographer] is a bridge from the sexually liberated 1970s to the more cautious 1990s, and Preston has walked much of that way as a standard-bearer to the cause for equal rights...." —*Library Journal*
"*My Life as a Pornographer*...is not pornography, but rather reflections upon the writing and production of it. In a deeply sex-phobic world, Preston has never shied away from a vision of the redemptive potential of the erotic drive. Better than perhaps anyone in our community, Preston knows how physical joy can bridge differences and make us well."
—*Lambda Book Report*

HUSTLING: A GENTLEMAN'S GUIDE TO THE FINE ART OF HOMOSEXUAL PROSTITUTION
$12.95/137-3

A must-read for any man who's ever considered selling IT, either to make ends meet, or just for fun. John Preston solicited the advice of "working boys" from across the country in his effort to produce the ultimate guide to the hustler's world.

"...fun and highly literary. What more could you expect from such an accomplished activist, author and editor?"
—*Drummer*

PAT CALIFIA
SENSUOUS MAGIC
$12.95/458-5

A new classic, destined to grace the shelves of anyone interested in contemporary sexuality.

"*Sensuous Magic* is clear, succinct and engaging even for the reader for whom S/M isn't the sexual behavior of choice.... When she is writing about the dynamics of sex and the technical aspects of it, Califia is the Dr. Ruth of the alternative sexuality set...."
—*Lambda Book Report*
"Finally, a 'how to' sex manual that doesn't involve new age mumbo jumbo or 'tricks' that require the agility of a Flying Wallenda.... Califia's strength as a writer lies in her ability to relay information without sounding condescending. If you don't understand a word or concept... chances are it's defined in the handy dictionary in the back...."
—*Futuresex*
"For either the uninitiated or the 'old-hand,' Califia is always a sexy delight to read."
—*Icon*
"One of the very best sex-manuals ever produced, and certainly the starting point for anyone at all interested in a complete overview of the scene and who wants to explore further or even just work their way back to base."
—*Divinity*
"Pat Califia's *Sensuous Magic* is a friendly, non-threatening, helpful guide and resource for 'adventurous couples' who are interested in expanding the erotic boundaries of their sexual relationships.... She captures the power of what it means to enter forbidden terrain, and to do so safely with someone else, and to explore the healing potential, spiritual aspects and the depth of S/M."
—*Bay Area Reporter*
"Don't take a dangerous trip into the unknown—buy this book and know where you're going!"
—*SKIN TWO*

MASQUERADE BOOKS

CARO SOLES, EDITOR
MELTDOWN! AN ANTHOLOGY OF EROTIC SCIENCE FICTION AND DARK FANTASY FOR GAY MEN
$12.95/203-5

Editor Caro Soles has put together one of the most explosive collections of gay erotic writing ever published. *Meltdown!* contains the very best examples of the increasingly popular sub-genre of erotic sci-fi/dark fantasy: stories meant to shock and delight, to send a shiver down the spine and start a fire down below.

LARS EIGHNER
ELEMENTS OF AROUSAL
$12.95/230-2

A guideline for success with one of publishing's best kept secrets: the novice-friendly field of gay erotic writing. Eighner details his craft, providing the reader with sure advice. Because that's what *Elements of Arousal* is all about: the application and honing of the writer's craft, which brought Eighner fame with not only the steamy *Bayou Boy*, but the illuminating *Travels with Lizbeth*.

STAN TAL, EDITOR
BIZARRE SEX
AND OTHER CRIMES OF PASSION
$12.95/213-2

From the pages of *Bizarre Sex*: Over twenty small masterpieces of erotic shock make this one of the year's most unexpectedly alluring anthologies. This incredible volume, edited by Stan Tal, includes such masters of erotic horror and fantasy as Edward Lee, Lucy Taylor and Nancy Kilpatrick.

MARCO VASSI
A DRIVING PASSION
$12.95/134-9

Marco Vassi was famous not only for his groundbreaking writing, but for the many lectures he gave regarding sexuality and the complex erotic philosophy he had spent much of his life working out. *A Driving Passion* collects the wit and insight Vassi brought to these lectures, and distills the philosophy that made him an underground sensation.

"The most striking figure in present-day American erotic literature. Alone among modern erotic writers, Vassi is working out a philosophy of sexuality."
—Michael Perkins, *The Secret Record*

"Vintage Vassi." —*Future Sex*

"An intriguing artifact... His eclectic quest for eroticism is somewhat poignant, and his fervor rarely lapses into silliness." —*Publishers Weekly*

THE EROTIC COMEDIES
$12.95/136-5

The Erotic Comedies marked a high point in Vassi's literary career. Short stories designed to shock and transform attitudes about sex and sexuality, *The Erotic Comedies* is both entertaining and challenging—and garnered Vassi some of the most lavish praise of his career. Also includes his groundbreaking writings on the Erotic Experience, including the concept of Metasex—the premise of which was derived from the author's own unbelievable experiences.

"To describe Vassi's writing as pornography would be to deny his very serious underlying purposes.... The stories are good, the essays original and enlightening, and the language and subject-matter intended to shock the prudish."—*Sunday Times* (UK)

"The comparison to [Henry] Miller is high praise indeed.... But reading Vassi's work, the analogy holds—for he shares with Miller an unabashed joy in sensuality, and a questing after experience that is the root of all great literature, erotic or otherwise.... Vassi was, by all accounts, a fearless explorer, someone who jumped headfirst into the world of sex, and wrote about what he found. And as he himself was known to say on more than one occasion, 'The most erotic organ is the mind.'"
—David L. Ulin, *The Los Angeles Reader*

THE SALINE SOLUTION
$12.95/180-2

"I've always read Marco's work with interest and I have the highest opinion not only of his talent but his intellectual boldness." —Norman Mailer

The story of one couple's spiritual crises during an age of extraordianry freedom. While renowned for his sexual philosophy, Vassi also experienced success in with fiction; *The Saline Solution* was one of the high points of his career, while still addressing the issue of sexuality.

THE STONED APOCALYPSE
$12.95/132-2

"...Marco Vassi is our champion sexual energist."
—*VLS*

During his lifetime, Marco Vassi was hailed as America's premier erotic writer. His reputation was worldwide. *The Stoned Apocalypse* is Vassi's autobiography, financed by his other groundbreaking erotic writing. Chronicling a cross-country roadtrip, *The Stoned Apocalypse* is rife with Vassi's insight into the American character and libido. One of the most vital portraits of "the 60s," this volume is a fitting testament to the writer's talents, and the sexual imagination of his generation.